CT Teaching Manual

eme

Before you begin, you should read the **Intructions to Users** on the facing infold. They will help you make the most of all the practical aspects of the book, for example finding a particular stucture, and will enable you to optimize your learning efforts. The manual contains a system of numbered legends to consult when you are repeating a chapter or simply brushing up your knowledge. Each chapter closes with several **Test Yourself!** questions, the answers to which are at the back of the book. Most CT images are accompanied by a gray scale sketch that indicates the type of tissue or organ according to the following examples:

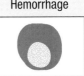

Schemata for CT Drawings:

All the drawings have been done according to the same gray scale. Air or gas, regardless of where they are found, are black; bone is white. Between these extremes, the shading varies for tissues, organs, and abnormalities independent of the image display settings. In addition, abnormalities such as metastases can be recognized by their specific patterns.

Parenchyma of larger organs (medium gray)

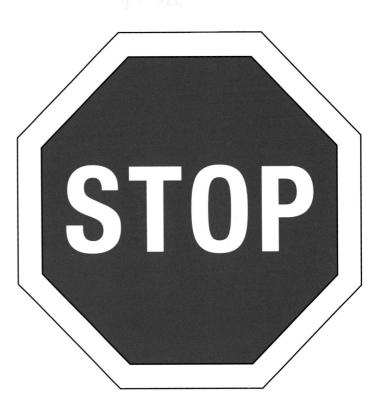

Air (black)

in the trachea

in the colon

Fat / CSF (almost black)

Small intestine (thin walls)

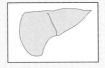
with G-I contents   with some CM   dense CM

Muscle (dark gray)

transverse section

longitudinal section

Bone (white)

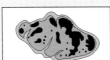
trabeculae

cortical

Colon with fecal residue and gas

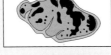

Lymph node (medium gray)

Blood vessels (light gray)

transverse section   Longitudinal section

Pancreas, salivary glands

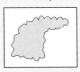

Brain parenchyma

Hemorrhage

Metastases

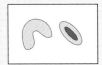

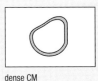

Library of Congress Cataloging-in-Publication Data is available from the publisher.

Important Note: Medicine is an ever-changing science undergoing continual development. Research and clinical experience are continually expanding our knowledge, in particular our knowledge of proper treatment and drug therapy. Insofar as this book mentions any dosage or application, readers may rest assured that the authors, editors, and publishers have made every effort to ensure that such references are in accordance with *the state of konwledge at the time of production of the book.*

Nevertheless this does not involve, imply, or express any guarantee or responsibility on the part of the publishers in respect of any dosage instructions and forms of application stated in the book. *Every user is requested to examine carefully* the manufacturers' leaflets accompanying each drug and to check, if necessary in consultation with a physician or specialist, whether the dosage schedules mentioned therein or the contraindications stated by the manufacturers differ from the statements made in the present book. Such examination is particularly important with drugs that are either rarely used or have been newly released on the market. Every dosage schedule or every form of application used is entirely at the user's own risk and responsibility. The authors and publishers request every user to report to the publishers any discrepancies or inaccuracies noticed.

Matthias Hofer, M.D.

Institute for Diagnostic Radiology
(Head: U. Mödder, M. D.)
Heinrich-Heine University
Düsseldorf, Germany

© 2000 Georg Thieme Verlag,
Rüdigerstraße 14, D-70469 Stuttgart, Germany
Thieme New York, 333 Seventh Avenue,
New York, N.Y. 10001 U.S.A.

Typesetting by Körner Offsetdruck, Düsseldorf

Printed in Germany by Körner Offsetdruck, Düsseldorf

ISBN 3-13-124351-1 (GTV)
ISBN 0-86577-897-3 (TNY)

Some of the product names, patents, and registered designs referred to in this book are in fact registered trademarks or proprietary names even though specific reference to this fact is not always made in the text. Therefore, the appearance of a name without designation as proprietary is not to be construed as a representation by the publisher that it is in the public domain.

Human anatomy has not changed much over the past millennia, but our way of looking at it has altered dramatically during the past few decades. Physicians and medical students have always needed a good topographical understanding of anatomy before seeing a patient. Nowadays this need is even greater. The cross-sectional images of ultrasound, MRI, and CT can only be interpreted with a clear understanding of anatomy. The Teaching Manual provides an ideal link between the classical approach to learning anatomy and the anatomical information revealed by the new imaging techniques.

The Manual has been designed to facilitate the learning of both cross-sectional anatomy and CT. Anatomical variations and pathologic findings are introduced in a clear and logical manner. The principles and practice of CT are presented without confusing terminology. This edition includes a description of spiral (helical) acquisitions and emphasizes the role of 3D display. The Manual addresses applications in all body areas and is richly illustrated with images of a wide range of diseases. The increasing utility of CT in diagnosis is a core feature in the Manual which will be of great value to medical students and residents. The Manual will also be a welcome refresher for more experienced clinicians.

The fact that the German edition of the Teaching Manual has already appeared in its second revised and expanded version indicates that it continues to be a complete success. We hope that this edition will also meet the needs of medical students and residents undergoing training in English speaking countries.

Düsseldorf, Summer 1999

Kristina Rascher and Niall Moore

Düsseldorf and Oxford

Abbreviations for texts:

3D	three dimensional	FNH	focal nodular hyperplasia of the liver	NHL	non-Hodgkin lymphoma
A., Aa.	artery, arteries	Gb	gallbladder	p.i.	post injection
a., ant.	anterior	GIT	gastrointestinal tract	pixel	picture element
a.p.	anteroposterior	HCC	hepatocellular carcinoma	PPI	parenchyma-pyelon index
amp.	ampule	HRCT	high resolution CT	PRIND	prolonged, reversible, ischemic
ao	aorta	HU	Hounsfield unit(s)		neurological deficit
AR	area = size of an ROI in cm^2	i.m.	intramuscular	Proc.	processus, process
b.w.	body weight	i.v.	intravenous	ROI	region of interest
BC	bronchial carcinoma	IUCD	intrauterine contraceptive device	SAH	subarachnoid hemorrhage
Ca	carcinoma	IVU	intravenous urogram	SAS	subarachnoid space
CCT	cranial CT	kg	kilogram	s.c.	subcutaneous
CHD	coronary heart disease	Kt.	kidney transplant	SCT	spiral CT (helical CT)
ChE	cholecystectomy	LA	lower abdomen	SLE	systemic lupus erythematosus
cm	centimeter	lat.	lateral	SMA	superior mesenteric artery
CM	contrast medium	Lig.	ligament(s)	Tg	thyroid gland
CSF	cerebrospinal fluid	LN	lymph node	TIA	transient ischemic attack
CT	computed tomography	LV	lumbar vertebra	TV	thoracic vertebra
CV	cervical vertebra	M., Mm.	muscle, muscles	UA	Upper abdomen
d	diameter or day	MA	mid abdomen	Ub	urinary bladder
DD	differential diagnosis	me	mean	V., Vv.	Vein, veins
DIC	disseminated intravascular coagulopathy	med.	medial	Vol	Volume
d$_S$	section/slice thickness	MIP	maximum intensity projection	voxel	volume element
ECG	electrocardiogram	mm	millimeter		
ESWL	extracorporal shock wave lithotripsy	MPR	multiplanar reconstruction		
ERCP	endoscopic retrograde cholangio-pancreatography	MR(I)	magnetic resonance (imaging)		
		N., Nn.	nerve, nerves		

Table of Contents

Table of Contents

General Principles of CT

Computed tomography is a special type of x-ray procedure that involves the indirect measurement of the weakening, or attenuation, of x-rays at numerous positions located around the patient being investigated. Basically speaking, all we know is

● what leaves the x-ray tube,
● what arrives at the detector and
● the position of the x-ray tube and detector for each position.

Simply stated, everything else is deduced from this information. Most CT slices are oriented vertical to the body`s axis. They are usually called axial or transverse sections. For each section the x-ray tube rotates around the patient to obtain a preselected section thickness **(Fig. 6.1)**. Most CT systems employ the continuous rotation and fan beam design: with this design, the x-ray tube and detector are rigidly coupled and rotate continuously around the scan field while x-rays are emitted and detected. Thus, the x-rays, which have passed through the patient, reach the detectors on the opposite side of the tube. The fan beam opening ranges from 40° to 60°, depending on the particular system design, and is defined by the angle originating at the focus of the x-ray tube and extending to the outer limits of the detector array.

Typically, images are produced for each 360° rotation, permitting a high number of measurement data to be acquired and sufficient dose to be applied. While the scan is being performed, attenuation profiles, also referred to as samples or projections, are obtained. Attenuation profiles are really nothing other than a collection of the signals obtained from all the detector channels at a given angular position of the tube-detector unit. Modern CT systems **(Fig. 6.4.)** acquire approximately 1400 projections over 360°, or about four projections per degree. Each attenuation profile comprises the data obtained from about 1500 detector channels, about 30 channels per degree in case of a 50° fan beam. While the patient table is moving continuously through the gantry, a digital radiograph ("scanogramm" or "localizer", **Fig. 6.2**) is produced on which the desired sections can be planned. For a CT examination of the spine or the head, the gantry is angled to the optimal orientation **(Fig. 6.3)**.

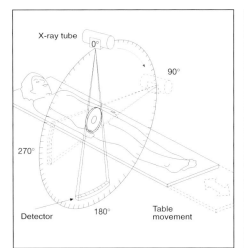

Fig. 6.1

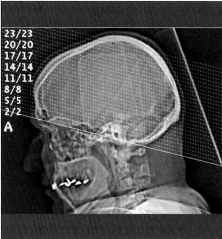

Fig. 6.2

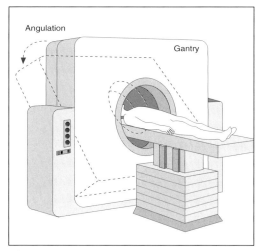

Fig. 6.3

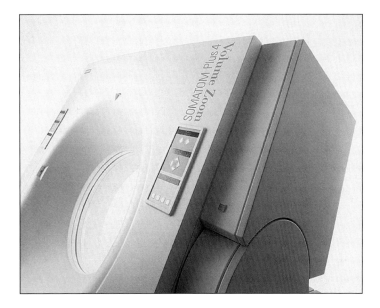

Fig. 6.4

The data obtained at the detector channel are passed on, profile for profile, to the detector electronics as electric signals corresponding to the actual x-ray attenuation. These electric signals are digitized and then transmitted to the image processor. At this stage, the images are reconstructed by means of the "pipeline principle", consisting of preprocessing, convolution, and back projection **(Fig. 7.1)**.

Preprocessing includes all the corrections taken to prepare the measured scan data for reconstruction, e.g., correction for dark current, dose output, calibration, channel correction, beam hardening, and spacing errors. These corrections are performed to further minimize the slight variations inherently found in the tube and detector components of the imaging chain.

Convolution is basically the use of negative values to correct for smearing inherent to simple back projection. If, for instance, a cylindric water phantom is scanned and reconstructed without convolution, the edges of this phantom will be extremely blurry **(Fig. 7.2a)**: What happens when just eight attenuation profiles of a small, highly absorbent cylindrical object are superimposed to create an image? Since the same part of the cylinder is measured by two overlapping projections, a star-shaped image is produced instead of what is in reality a cylinder. By introducing negative values just beyond the positive portion of the attenuation profiles, the edges of this cylinder can be sharply depicted **(Fig. 7.2b)**.

Back projection involves the reassigning of the convolved scan data to a 2D image matrix representing the section of the patient that is scanned. This is performed profile for profile for the entire image reconstruction process. The image matrix can be thought of as analogous to a chessboard, consisting of typically 512 x 512 or 1024 x 1024 picture elements, usually called "pixels". Back projection results in an exact density being assigned to each of these pixels, which are then displayed as a lighter or darker shade of gray. The lighter the shade of gray, the higher the density of the tissue within the pixel (e.g., bone).

The Influence of kV

When examining anatomic regions with higher absorption (e.g., CT of the head, shoulders, thoracic or lumbar spine, pelvis, and larger patients), it is often advisable to use higher kV levels in addition to, or instead of, higher mA values: when you choose higher kV, you are hardening the x-ray beam. Thus x-rays can penetrate anatomic regions with higher absorption more easily. As a positive side effect, the lower energy components of the radiation are reduced, which is desirable since low energy x-rays are absorbed by the patient and do not contribute to the image. For imaging of infants or bolus tracking, it may be advisable to utilize kV lower than the standard setting.

Scan Time

It is advantageous to select a scan time as short as possible, particularly in abdominal or chest studies where heart movement and peristalsis may degrade image quality. Other CT investigations can also benefit from fast scan times due to decreased probability of involuntary patient motion. On the other hand, it may be necessary to select a longer scan time to provide sufficient dose or to enable more samples for maximal spatial resolution. Some users may also consciously choose longer scan times to lower the mA setting and thus increase the likelihood of longer x-ray tube life.

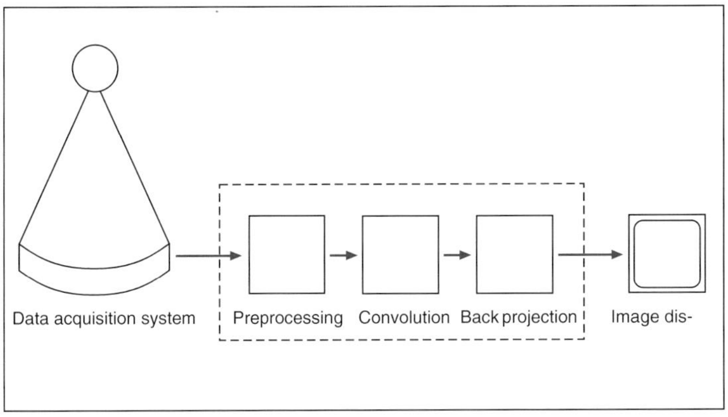

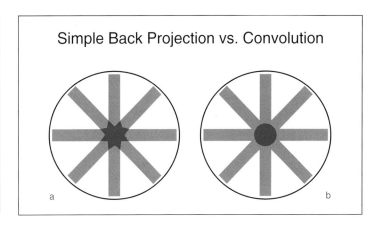

Fig. 7.1 The pipeline principle of image reconstruction

Fig. 7.2a Back projection without convolution

Fig. 7.2b Back projection with convolution

Slice Thickness

The decision between thinner and thicker slices is primarily determined by the desire to obtain a higher spatial resolution or more contrast detectability. When examining the inner ear we are most interested in getting the best possible spatial resolution to optimize the visualization of the inner ear's fine bony structures in contrast to the surrounding air. Therefore a slice thickness of less than 2 mm is selected. In many CT studies of the lung a high spatial resolution is also the dominating factor. In liver studies contrast detectability is of more importance, hence we use thick slices to optimize photon efficiency and maintain an acceptable noise level.

Conventional CT as Compared to Spiral or Helical CT

In conventional CT, a series of equally spaced images is acquired sequentially through a specific region, e.g. the abdomen or the head **(Fig. 8.1)**. There is a short pause after each section in order to advance the patient table to the next preset position. The section thickness and overlap/intersection gap are selected at the outset. The raw data for each image level is stored separately. The short pause between sections allows the conscious patient to breathe without causing major respiratory artifacts. However, the examination may take several minutes, depending on the body region and the size of the patient. Proper timing of image acquisition after i.v.

In SCT, images are acquired continuously while the patient table is advanced through the gantry. The x-ray tube describes an apparent helical path around the patient **(Fig. 8.2)**. If table advance is coordinated with the time required for a 360° rotation (pitch factor), data acquisition is complete and uninterrupted. This modern technique has greatly improved CT because respiratory artifacts and inconsistencies do not affect the single dataset as markedly as in conventional CT. The single dataset can be used to reconstruct slices of differing thickness or at differing intervals. Even overlapping slices can be reconstructed.

Data acquisition for the abdomen takes only 1–2 minutes: two or

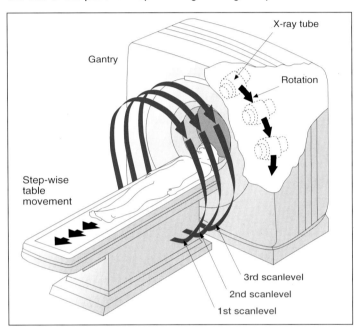

Fig. 8.1

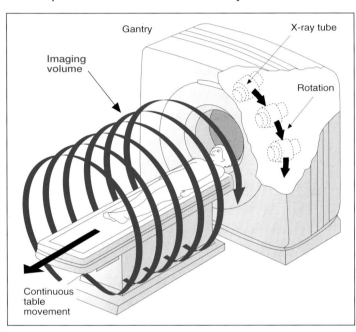

Fig. 8.2

contrast media is particularly important for assessing perfusion effects. CT is the technique of choice for acquiring complete 2D axial images of the body without the disadvantages of superimposed bone and/or air as seen in conventional x-ray images.

three helices, each about 25–30 seconds, are obtained. The time limit is determined by the duration a patient can hold his breath and the necessary cooling of the x-ray tubes. Image reconstruction takes longer. An assessment of renal function following CM will require a short break to allow for CM excretion to occur.

One of the advantages of the helical technique is that lesions smaller than the conventional thickness of a slice can be detected. Small liver metastases **(7)** will be missed if inconsistent depth of

respiration results in them not being included in the section **(Fig. 8.3a)**. The metastases would appear in overlapping reconstructions from the dataset of the helical technique **(Fig. 8.3b)**.

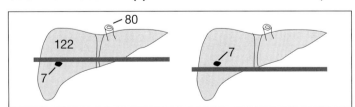

Fig. 8.3a Conventional CT

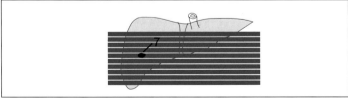

Fig. 8.3b Spiral CT

Four Slice Spiral CT

This newest technique has lead to the possibility of acquiring up to 80 mm of anatomy per second and reduces scan rotation time to 500 ms! These scanners combine the ability to use ultrathin slices down to 0.5 mm and to acquire large anatomic volumes. The basic hardware changes are found in the detector design. Instead of current fixed matrix detectors of uniform length with gaps or "dead space," the new adaptive array detectors entail detectors with different lengths along the z-axis, with the larger detectors toward the edge of the cone beam and thin slices in the center. Different combinations of the adjacent detectors improve scan speed, temporal and contrast resolution by a factor up to eight times that of conventional, single-slice, 1-second CT scanners.

When both liver and pancreas are included, many users prefer a reduced slice thickness from 10 mm to 3 mm to improve image sharpness. This increases, however, the noise level by approximately 80%. Therefore it would be necessary to employ 80% more mA or to lengthen the scan time (this increases the mAs product) to maintain image quality.

Pitch

Spiral users have an additional advantage: pitch is the ratio between table feed per rotation (not per second!) and slice thickness. In the spiral image reconstruction process, most of the data points were not actually measured in the particular slice being reconstructed **(Fig. 9.1)**. Instead, data are acquired outside this slice (●) and interpolated with more importance, or "contibution", being attached to the data located closest to the slice (X). In other words: The data point closest to the slice receives more weight, or counts more, in the reconstruction of an image at the desired table position.

This results in an interesting phenomenon. The patient dose (actually given in mGy) is determined by the mAs per rotation divided by the pitch, and the image dose is equal to the mAs per rotation without considering the pitch. If for instance 150 mAs per rotation with a pitch of 1.5 are employed, the patient dose in mGy is linear related to 100 mAs, and the image dose is related to 150

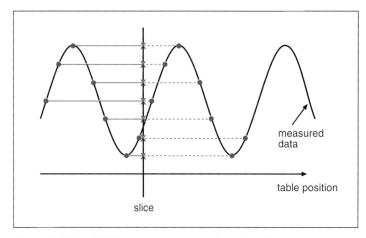

Fig. 9.1 Wide (360°) spiral reconstruction algorithm

mAs. Therefore spiral users can improve contrast detectability by selecting high mA values, increase the spatial resolution (image sharpness) by reducing slice thickness, and employ pitch to adjust the length of the spiral range as desired, all while reducing the patient's dose! More slices can be acquired without increasing the dose or stressing the x-ray tube.

This technique is especially helpful when data are reformatted to create other 2D views, like sagittal, oblique, coronal, or 3D views (MIP, surface shaded imaging, see pp. 16/17).

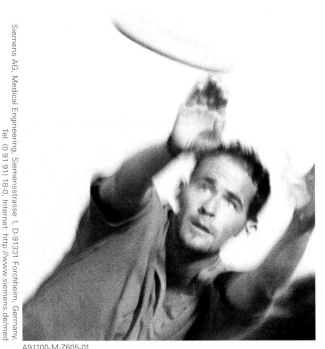
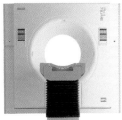

Anatomic Orientation

An image on the display is not only a 2D representation of anatomy, it contains information about the mean attenuation of tissue in a matrix consisting of about 512 x 512 elements (**pixels**). A section (**Fig. 10.1**) has a defined thickness (d_S) and is composed of a matrix of cubic or cuboid units (**voxels**) of identical size. This technical aspect is the reason for the partial volume effects explained below. An image is usually displayed as if the body were viewed from caudal. Thus the right side of the patient is on the left side of the image and vice versa (**Fig. 10.1**). For example, the liver (**122**) is located in the right half of the body, but appears in the left half of the image. Organs of the left side such as the stomach (**129**) and the spleen (**133**) appear on the right half of an image. Anterior aspects of the body, for example the abdominal wall, are repre-

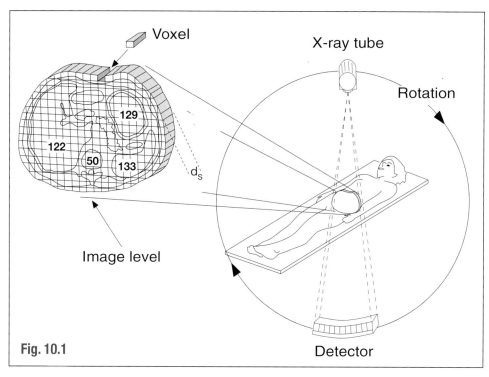

Fig. 10.1

sented in the upper parts of an image, posterior aspects such as the spine (**50**) are lower. With this system CT images are more easily compared with conventional x-rays.

Partial Volume Effects

The radiologist determines the thickness of the image (d_S). 8–10 mm is usually chosen for thoracic or abdominal examinations, and 2–5 mm for the skull, spine, orbits, or petrosal bones. A structure may therefore be included in the entire thickness of a slice (**Fig. 10.2a**) or in only a part of it (**Fig. 10.3a**). The gray scale value of a voxel depends on the mean attenuation of all structures within it. If a structure has a regular shape within a section, it will appear well defined. This is the case for the abdominal aorta (**89**) and the inferior vena cava (**80**) shown in **Figures 10.2a, b**.

Partial volume effects occur when structures do not occupy the entire thickness of a slice, for example when a section includes part of a vertebral body (**50**) and part of a disk (**50e**) the anatomy will be poorly defined (**Figs. 10.3a, b**). This is also true if an organ tapers within a section as seen in **Figures 10.4a, b**. This is the reason for the poor definition of the renal poles or the borders of the gallbladder (**126**) or urinary bladder.

Artifacts caused by breathing during image acquisition are discussed on page 17.

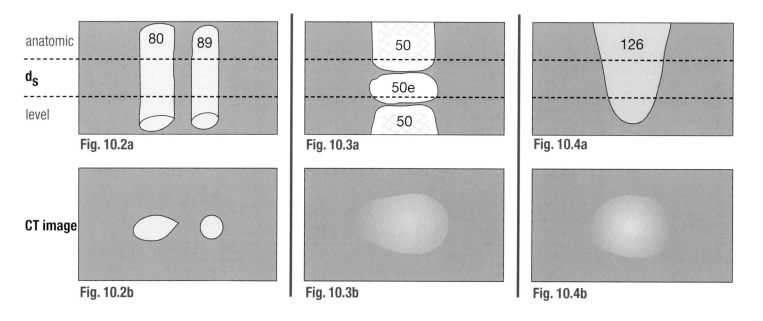

Fig. 10.2a

Fig. 10.3a

Fig. 10.4a

Fig. 10.2b

Fig. 10.3b

Fig. 10.4b

Distinguishing between Nodular and Tubular Structures

It is essential to differentiate between possibly enlarged or affected LNs and vessels or muscles which have been cut in transverse section. This may be extremely difficult in a single image because these structures have similar density values (gray tones). One should therefore always analyze adjacent cranial and caudal images and compare the structures in question to determine whether they are nodular swellings or continue as more or less tubular structures (**Fig. 11.1**): A lymph node (**6**) will appear in only one or two slices and cannot be traced in adjacent images (compare **Figs. 11.1a, b,** and **c**). The aorta (**89**) or the inferior cava (**80**), or a muscle, for example the iliopsoas (**31**), can be traced through a cranio-caudal series of images.

If there is a suspicious nodular swelling in one image it should become an automatic reaction to compare adjacent levels to clarify whether it is simply a vessel or muscle in cross-section. This procedure will also enable quick identification of the partial volume effects described on the previous page.

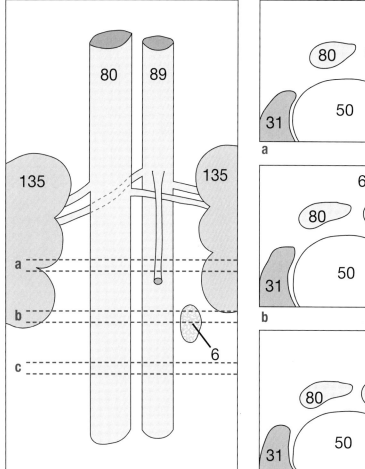

Fig. 11.1

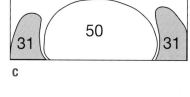

Densitometry (Measurement of Density)

If it is uncertain, for example, whether fluid found in the pleural cavity is a pleural effusion or a hemothorax, a measurement of the liquid's density will clarify the differential diagnosis. The same applies to focal lesions in the parenchyma of the liver or the kidney. However, it is not advisable to carry out measurements of single voxels (=volume element, see **Fig. 10.1**) since such data are liable to statistical fluctuations which can make the attenuation unreliable. It is more accurate to position a larger "region of interest" (ROI) consisting of several voxels in a focal lesion, a structure, or an amount of fluid. The computer calculates the mean density levels of all voxels and also provides the standard deviation (SD).

One must be particularly careful not to overlook beam-hardening artifacts (**Fig. 15.2**) or partial volume effects. If a mass does not extend through the entire thickness of a slice, measurements of density will include the tissue next to it (**Figs. 117.2** and **127.1–127.3**). The density of a mass will be measured correctly only if it fills the entire thickness of the slice (d_S) (**Fig. 11.2**). It is then more likely that measurements will only the mass (hatched

area in **Fig. 11.2a**). If d_S is greater than the mass's diameter, for example a small lesion in an unfavorable position, it can only appear in partial volume at any scan level (**Fig. 11.2b**).

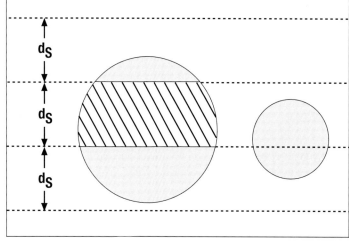

Fig. 11.2   a   b

Density Levels of Different Types of Tissues

Modern equipment has a capacity of 4096 gray tones, which represent different density levels in HUs. The density of water was arbitrarily set at 0 HU and that of air at –1000 HU **(Table 12.1a)**. The monitor can display a maximum of 256 gray tones. However, the human eye is able to discriminate only approximately 20. Since the densities of human tissues extend over a fairly narrow range (a window) of the total spectrum **(Table 12.1b)**, it is possible to select a window setting to represent the density of the tissue of interest.

The mean density level of the window should be set as close as possible to the density level of the tissue to be examined. The lung, with its high air content, is best examined at a low HU window setting **(Fig. 13.1c)**, whereas bones require an adjustment to high levels **(Fig. 13.2c)**. The width of the window influences the contrast of the images: the narrower the window, the greater the contrast since the 20 gray tones cover only a small scale of densities.

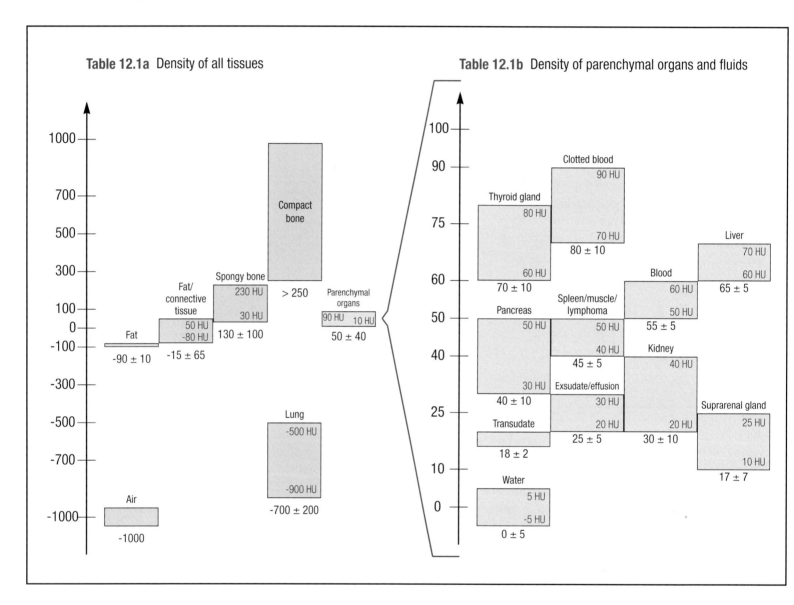

Table 12.1a Density of all tissues

Table 12.1b Density of parenchymal organs and fluids

It is noteworthy that the density levels of almost all soft-tissue organs lie within a narrow range between 10 and 90 HUs **(Table 12.1b)**. The only exception is the lung and, as mentioned above, this requires a special window setting **(Figs. 13.1a–c)**. With respect to hemorrhages, it should be taken into account that the density level of recently coagulated blood lies about 30 HU above that of fresh blood. This density drops again in older hemorrhages or liquefied thromboses. An exudate with a protein content above 30 g/l cannot be readily distinguished from a transudate (protein content below 30 g/l) at conventional window settings. In addition, the high degree of overlap between the densities of, for example, lymphomas, spleen, muscles, and pancreas makes it clear that it is not possible to deduce, from density levels alone, what substance or tissue is present.

Finally, standard density values also fluctuate between individuals, depending as well on the amount of CM in the circulating blood and in the organs. The latter aspect is of particular importance for the examination of the urogenital system, since i.v. CM is rapidly excreted by the kidney, resulting in rising density levels in the parenchyma during the scanning procedure. This effect can be put to use when judging kidney function (see **Fig. 129.1**).

Documentation of Different Windows

When the images have been acquired, a hard copy is printed for documentation. For example: in order to examine the mediastinum and the soft tissues of the thoracic wall, the window is set such that muscles **(13, 14, 20–26)**, vessels **(89, 90, 92...)**, and fat are clearly represented in shades of gray. The soft-tissue window **(Fig. 13.1a)** is centered at 50 HU with a width of about 350 HU. The result is a representation of density values from −125 HU (50–350/2) up to +225 HU (50 + 350/2). All tissues with a density lower than −125 HU, such as the lung, are represented in black. Those with density levels above +225 appear white and their internal structural features cannot be differentiated.

If lung parenchyma is to be examined, for example when scanning for nodules, the window center will be lower at about −200 HU, and the window wider (2000 HU). Low-density pulmonary structures **(96)** can be much more clearly differentiated in this so-called lung window **(Fig. 13.1c)**.

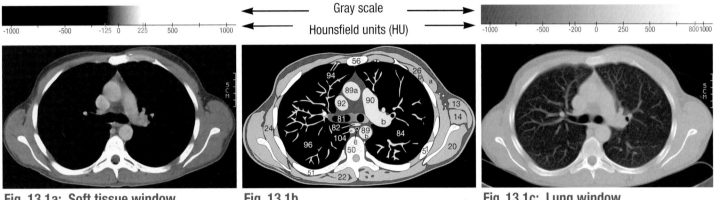

Gray scale

Hounsfield units (HU)

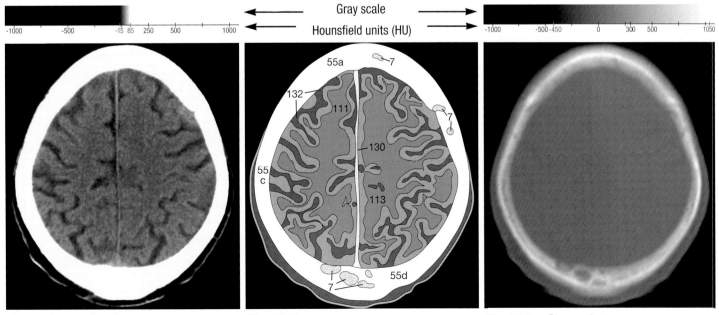

Fig. 13.1a: Soft tissue window Fig. 13.1b Fig. 13.1c: Lung window

In order to achieve maximal contrast between gray and white matter in the brain, it is necessary to select a special brain window because the density values of gray and white matter differ only slightly. The brain window must be very narrow (80 to 100 HU => high contrast) and the center must lie close to the mean density of cerebral tissue (35 HU) to demonstrate these slight differences **(Fig. 13.2a)**. At this setting it is of course impossible to examine the skull since all structures hyperdense to 75–85 HU appear white. The bone window should therefore have a much higher center, at about +300 HU, and a sufficient width of about 1500 HU. The metastases **(7)** in the occipital bone **(55d)** would only be visible in the appropriate bone window **(Fig. 13.2c)**, but not in the brain window **(Fig. 13.2a)**. On the other hand, the brain is practically invisible in the bone window; small cerebral metastases would not be detected. One must always be aware of these technical aspects, especially since hard copies are not usually printed at each window setting. The examiner should review thoroughly the images on the screen in additional windows to avoid missing important pathologic features. Examination of the liver poses special problems and is dealt with separately on page 116.

Gray scale

Hounsfield units (HU)

Fig. 13.2a: Brain window Fig. 13.2b Fig. 13.2c: Bone window

Medical History

Prior to any CT examination, an assessment of the medical history and laboratory results must be carried out. Among other data on the request card, it is important to note whether the patient has already undergone CT so that the new images can be compared with the earlier ones. Information about previous surgery and radiotherapy in the region to be covered by CT is also important as well as results of previous x-ray examinations. It is much more difficult to make a differential diagnosis if the radiologist is not informed about these aspects of the past medical history.

Renal Function

Unless the only indication for CT is to determine the precise location of a fracture (for example of a facial bone), most examinations require the i.v. administration of an iodine-containing CM. Since CM is excreted by the kidneys and may reduce the tubular function [8], the physician should evaluate the patient's renal function by measuring the plasma creatinine prior to CT. If there are signs of incipient renal failure, CM should only be given in a very narrow range of indications [9, 10]. Diabetic patients on biguanid therapy must be given special attention [8, 9]. CM may cause lactic acidosis, induce chronic reduction of renal function, or aggravate renal insufficiency. Until recently, in cases where CM was absolutely necessary for a dialysis patient, the CT examination was scheduled so that dialysis followed immediately. Recent reports, however, show that it is not necessary for dialysis to follow immediately [11] and that there are no complications if the CM circulates for a day or two until the next dialysis.

Creatinine levels can be checked quickly and at low cost; it should be routine practice. Including the result on the request card saves time.

Hyperthyroidism

Examining for hyperthyroidism is costly and time-consuming. Nevertheless, the referring physician must exclude thyroid hyperactivity or an autonomous nodule if there is a clinical suspicion of hyperthyroidism before a CT examination involving CM is carried out. Laboratory parameters, sonography, and possibly scintigraphy may be necessary. In other cases, the information "no clinical evidence of hyperthyroidism" or even better, the documentation of thyroid function on the request card is helpful. Thus, the radiologist can be sure that testing has been done.

Note that reference values may vary from one laboratory to another. Some determine the absolute T_3 or T_4 levels, others free T_3 or T_4 and the units and reference values may be different. Check with your laboratory which units and normal ranges are valid if these are not included on the report. The risk of a thyroid crisis caused by the iodine-containing CM may be avoided. If radioiodine therapy for hyperthyroidism is planned, the i.v. application of CM could lead to a saturation of the iodine uptake system in the thyroid gland. Radioiodine therapy would have to be delayed for some time as a result.

Table 14.1 Normal thyroid hormone levels

TSH:	0.23 – 4.0 µg/ml		
TT_3:	0.8 – 1.8 ng/ml	TT_4:	45 –115 ng/ml
FT_3:	3.5 – 6.0 pg/ml	FT_4:	8.0 – 20.0 pg/ml

Adverse Reactions to Contrast Media

Ever since nonionic CM were introduced at the end of the 1970s, adverse reactions have only rarely be encountered [12–14]. Nevertheless, previous reactions to CM should be excluded in the patient's medical history. The severity of any reaction to CM in the past is of great importance. If the patients give a history of itching or hives following an angiogram, venogram or i.v. pyelogram, or after a previous CT examination with CM, premedication adjusted to the individual case is advisable. With a history of hypotension or cardiovascular collapse, CM should not be given or only after thorough reassessment of the clinical indication and appropriate premedication. As a general rule, patients who require premedication because of a previous reaction should be kept NPO prior to the examination. This reduces the danger of aspiration of gastric contents in cases with severe reactions that require intubation and ventilation.

Premedication in Cases of Suspected Previous Adverse Reactions to Contrast Media

In cases of mild adverse reactions, premedication is accomplished with H_1 and H_2 receptor antagonists, possibly combined with a low dosage of a rapidly acting steroid. The dosage is calculated according to body weight. Premedication should be carried out intravenously 1–2 hours prior to the CM injection, slowly and in separate ampules (!) in order to prevent any CM-induced allergic histamine release. Side effects such as raised intraocular pressure or urinary retention may occur. In addition, drowsiness may occur for about 8 hours following administration of these drugs so driving must be avoided for this period. Patients with obstructive glaucoma or those with benign prostatic hypertrophy must be given special attention. If an outpatient CT examination is scheduled, the patient must be informed about reduced drowsiness and the possibility of temporarily impaired vision; he or she should be accompanied on the way home.

You will find checklists of all key words concerning medical histories and suggestions for premedication on a practical card in the rear foldout.

Oral Administration of Contrast Medium

After a period of fasting, liquid CM should be drunk in small portions over a period of 30–60 minutes before the CT examination starts so that the entire GIT is completely opacified. The patient should therefore arrive at least 1 hour before an abdominal CT examination. In order to facilitate the correct choice of CM, the radiologist must be informed on the request card whether surgery is planned shortly after CT or whether there is any suspicion of perforation or fistula (see also p. 18). In such cases water-soluble gastrografin would be used instead of a CM containing barium sulfate. And finally, where possible, CT of the abdomen should be delayed for 3 days after a conventional barium examination has been carried out (for example: barium swallow, barium meal, small bowl enema, barium enema). Usually, the digital projection radiograph (scanogram **Fig. 15.1a**, scout view) would show that residual barium in the GIT would result in major artifacts **(Fig. 15.1b)**, rendering CT valueless. The sequence of diagnostic procedures for patients with abdominal diseases should therefore be carefully planned.

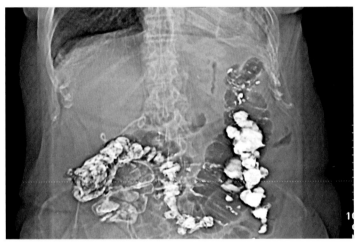

Fig. 15.1a

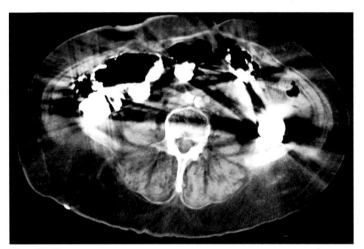

Fig. 15.1b

Informing the Patient

Understandably, patients have doubts about the harmful effects of the x-ray burden involved in CT. Worries can usually be reduced if you relate diagnostic x-ray exposure to natural background radiation. Naturally, the patient must have the feeling that he or she is being taken seriously and his or her worries are understood, otherwise confidence and trust in the radiologist are threatened. Many patients are relieved to know that they can communicate with the radiographers in the control room via an intercom and that the examination can be interrupted or terminated at any time if there are unexpected problems.

Patients with claustrophobia may feel more comfortable if they close their eyes during the examination; the close proximity of the gantry is then less of a problem. In very rare cases, a mild sedative may be helpful.

Removal of all Metallic Objects

Naturally, jewelry of any kind and removable dental prostheses must be removed before the head or neck are examined in order to avoid artifacts. In **Figures 15.2a** and **b** the effects of such artifacts **(3)** are obvious. Only the cervical vertebral body **(50)** and the adjacent vessels **(86)** are defined; the other structures are unrecognizable. For the same reason all clothing with metallic hooks, buttons, or zippers should be removed before thoracic or abdominal CTs are performed.

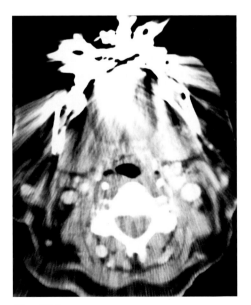

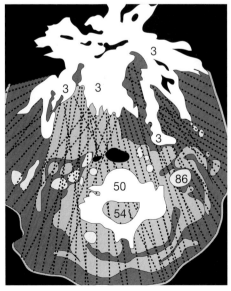

Fig. 15.2a

Fig. 15.2b

3D Reconstructions

Because the helical or spiral technique acquires a continuous, single volume dataset for an entire body region, imaging of fractures and blood vessels has improved markedly. Several different methods of 3D reconstruction have become established:

Maximal Intensity Projection

MIP is a mathematical method that extracts hyperintense voxels from 2D or 3D datasets [6, 7]. These voxels are selected from several different angles through the dataset and then projected as a 2D image (**Fig. 16.1**). A 3D impression is acquired by altering the projection angle in small steps and then viewing the reconstructed images in quick succession (i.e., in cine mode). This procedure is also used for examining contrast-enhanced blood vessels.

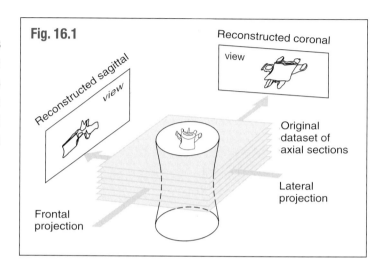

Fig. 16.1

Multiplanar Reconstruction

This technique makes it possible to reconstruct coronal and sagittal as well as oblique planes. MPR has become a valuable tool in the diagnosis of fractures and other orthopedic indications. For example, conventional axial sections do not always provide enough information about fractures. A good example is the undisplaced hairline fracture (✷) without cortical discontinuity that can be more effectively demonstrated by MPR (**Fig. 16.2a**).

3D Surface Shaded Display

This method shows the surface of an organ or a bone that has been defined in Hounsfield units above a particular threshold value. The angle of view, as well as the location of a hypothetical source of light (from which the computer calculates shadowing) are crucial for obtaining optimal reconstructions. The fracture of the distal radius shown in the MPR in **Figure 16.2a** is seen clearly in the bone surface in **Figure 16.2b**.

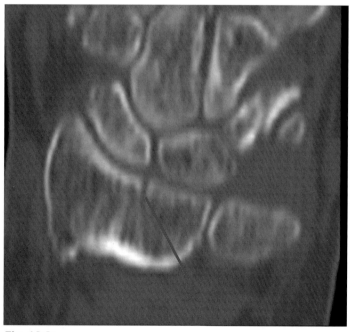

Fig. 16.2a

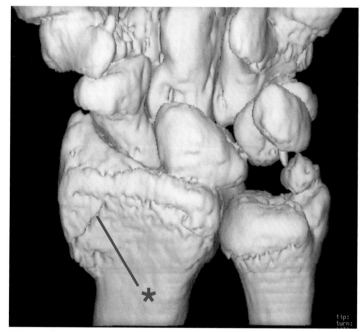

Fig. 16.2b

(**Figs. 16.2a** and **16.2b** supplied with the kind permission of J. Brackins Romero, M. D., Recklinghausen)

3D surface shaded displays are also valuable in planning surgery as in the case of the traumatic injury to the spinal column seen in **Figures 17a, b,** and **c**. Since the angle of view can be freely determined, the thoracic compression fracture (✷) and the state of the intervertebral foramina can be examined from several different angles (anterior in **Fig. 17.1a** and lateral in **Fig. 17.1b**). The sagittal MPR in **Figure 17.1c** determines whether any bone fragments have become dislocated into the spinal canal (compare with myelography CT on page 147).

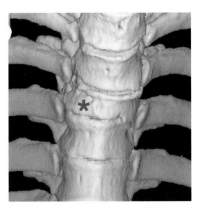

Fig. 17.1a

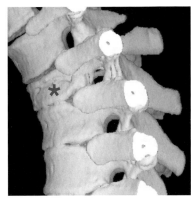

Fig. 17.1b

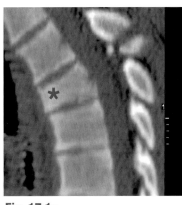

Fig. 17.1c

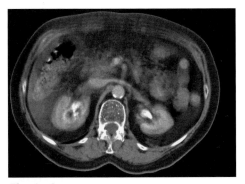

Fig. 17.2

Respiration

Before starting the examination, the patient should be told of the need for controlled breathing. For conventional CT, the patient is instructed to breathe before each new image acquisition and then to hold his or her breath for a few seconds. In the helical technique it is necessary to stop breathing for about 20–30 seconds. If the patient cannot comply, diaphragmatic movement will lead to image blur with a marked deterioration in image quality (Fig. 17.2). In the case of neck examinations, swallowing influences the quality of the images more than breathing

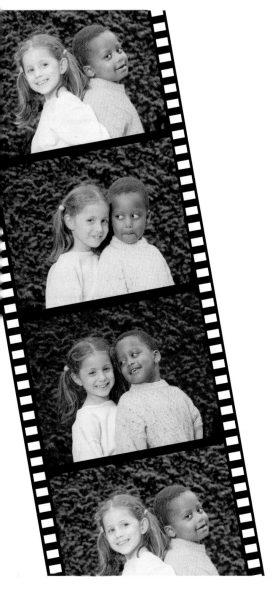
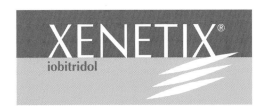
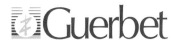

Oral Administration of Contrast Media

For CT examination of the abdomen and pelvis, it is of major advantage to be able to readily differentiate the GIT from adjacent muscles or other organs. This can be accomplished by opacifying the intestinal lumen with an orally administered CM. For example, without CM it is difficult to distinguish between the duodenum (**130**) and the head of the pancreas (**131** in **Fig. 18.1**). Equally, other parts of the intestinal tract (**140**) would also be very similar to neighboring structures. After an oral CM, both the duodenum and the pancreas can be well delineated (**Fig. 18.2a, b**). In order to acquire images of optimal quality, the patient should fast (be NBM) before drinking CM.

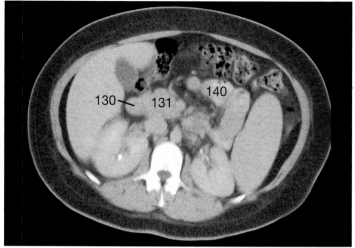

Fig. 18.1

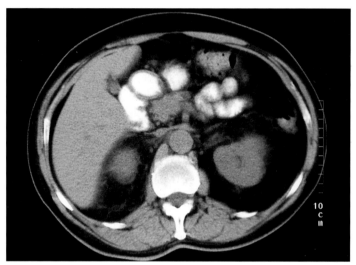

Fig. 18.2a

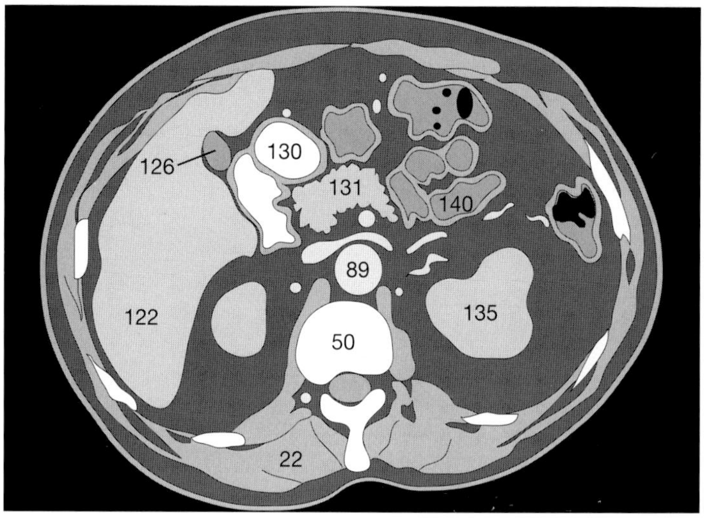

Fig. 18.2b

Choice of the Appropriate Contrast Media

The best coating of the mucous membranes is achieved with barium sulfate; however, this is not water soluble. This oral CM should therefore not be used if abdominal surgery involving opening of the bowel lumen is scheduled, such as in partial resections or anastomotic sutures, or if there is any risk of injury to the bowel. Neither should barium sulfate be used in cases of a suspected fistula or a GIT perforation. A watersoluble CM, such as gastrografin is then employed; it can be resorbed by the body after it spreads into the abdominal cavity.

For an optimal assessment of the stomach walls, plain water is increasingly used as a hypodense CM in combination with intravenous buscopan, which relaxes the muscularis [15, 16].

If the urinary bladder has been removed and an ilial conduit constructed, the abdomen is examined first with an intravenous CM which is excreted into the urine in the conduit but not within the native intestines. If necessary, the intestines can be examined in a second scan after oral CM.

The Time Factor

To opacify the proximal parts of the GIT, a period of about 20–30 min is sufficient; the patient swallows the CM in several small portions. However, if the entire colon and especially the rectum need to be opacified with barium sulfate, a period of at least 45–60 min is necessary in a fasting patient. The watersoluble CM gastrografin spreads somewhat more rapidly. For the pelvic organs (bladder, cervix, or ovary), 100–200 ml of CM may be given rectally to insure that tumors are clearly differentiated from the lower intestinal tract.

Dosage

To achieve complete opacification of the entire GIT, 250–300 ml of a barium sulfate suspension are dissolved and thoroughly mixed with water (1000 ml). For adequate contrast of the entire GIT, 10–20 ml of water-soluble gastrografin (in 1000 ml of water) are enough.

If only the upper part of the GIT needs to be opacified, 500 ml of either medium are sufficient.

Intravenous Contrast Media

An increase in the density of blood vessels not only demarcates them better from muscles and organs but also provides information on the rate of blood perfusion (CM uptake) in pathologically altered tissues: disturbances of the blood-brain barrier, the borders of abscesses, or the inhomogeneous uptake of CM in tumorlike lesions are only a few examples. This phenomenon is called contrast enhancement, i.e. the density is increased by the CM and thus the signal intensified.

Depending upon the question being asked, an unenhanced (plain) scan should be obtained before injecting the CM intravenously. Vascular grafts, inflammatory processes in bone, as well as abscess walls are more easily diagnosed if unenhanced images can be compared with contrast-enhanced images. The same holds true for focal liver lesions examined using conventional CT techniques. If helical CT is available, a series of liver images in the early phase of arterial CM perfusion followed by a series in the phase of venous drainage [17] would be obtained instead of unenhanced images. This procedure makes it possible to detect even small focal lesions (see p. 116).

Preparing the i.v. Line

The CM is injected intravenously, and the bolus becomes longer and diluted as it passes through the pulmonary circulation. The injection should therefore ideally have a rapid flow rate of 2–6 ml/sec for achieving sufficient density enhancement of the vessels [18]. A Venflon canula with a diameter of at least 1.0 mm (20G), or preferably 1.2–1.4 mm (18G–17G), is used. Checking that the canula is correctly sited in the vessel is very important. A trial injection of sterile saline at a high flow rate into the vein should be carried out before injecting CM. The absence of subcutaneous swelling confirms proper positioning; the fact that the vein can accommodate the intended flow can also be confirmed.

Dosage

Dosage is calculated on the basis of b.w. and according to the diagnostic question at hand: examinations of the neck or of an aortic aneurysm (for example in order to exclude the presence of a dissection flap), require higher concentrations than cranial CTs. When tolerance to CM and optimal vessel contrast are balanced, a dosage of, for example, 1.2 ml/kg b.w. at a concentration of 0.623 g Iopromid/ml (ULTRAVIST 300) provides good results.

Inflow Phenomena

The streaming artifact of enhanced and unenhanced blood results from a short interval between the start of injection and the onset of data acquisition. Since inflow is usually from one side via the axillary, subclavian, and brachiocephalic veins (91) into the superior vena cava (92), there is an apparent filling defect within the vena cava (Figs. 19.1a–19.3b). Knowing about such inflow phenomena avoids a false positive diagnosis of venous thrombosis. Using too high concentrations of CM in this area could result in disturbing artifacts, especially with the helical technique (Fig. 21.3a). More inflow phenomena will be described on the next pages.

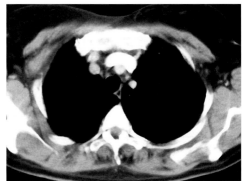

Fig. 19.1a

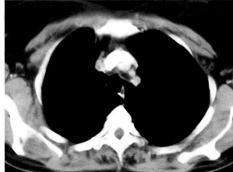

Fig. 19.2a

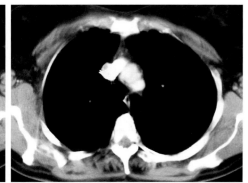

Fig. 19.3a

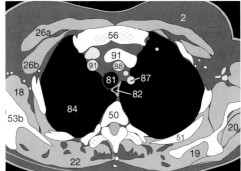

Fig. 19.1b

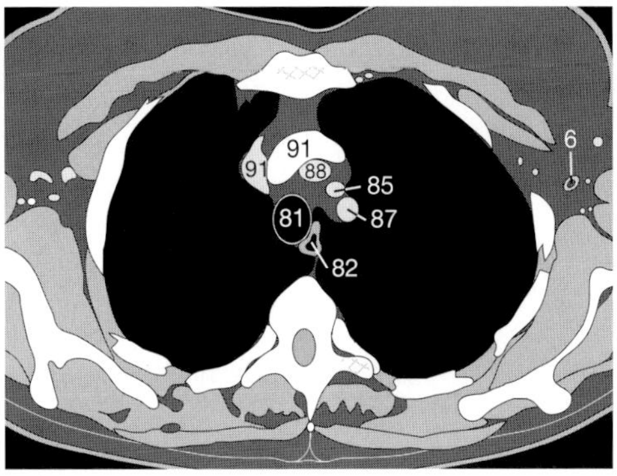

Fig. 19.2b

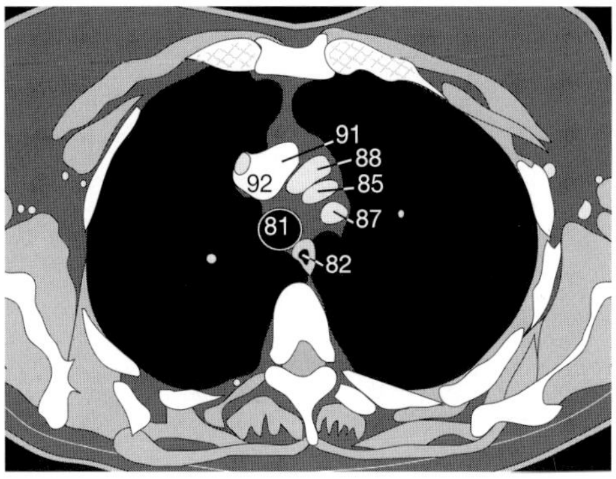

Fig. 19.3b

Application of Contrast Media

Flow phenomena can also be seen in the inferior vena cava **(80)** at the level of the renal veins **(111)**. These veins may contain blood which has a fairly high concentration of CM and this blood mixes with unenhanced blood returning from the lower extremities and pelvic organs. In the early post-contrast phase the vena cava **(80)** caudal to the level of the renal veins is hypodense relative to the adjacent aorta **(89)** as in **Figures 20.1a, b**.

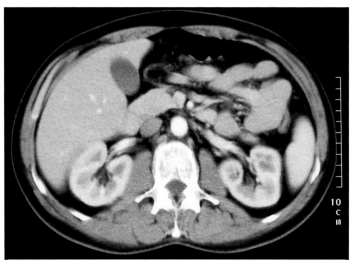

Fig. 20.1a

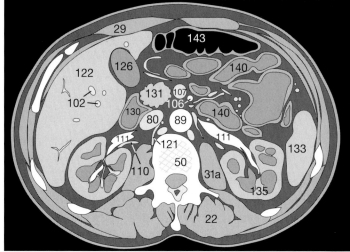

Fig. 20.1b

Immediately above the renal veins, the contents of the inferior vena cava may appear bilaterally enhanced by the blood from the kidneys whereas the central part is still unenhanced **(Fig. 20.2a, b)**. If the renal veins do not empty into the cava at the same level or if a kidney has been removed, a unilateral enhancement may occur **(Fig. 20.3a, b)**. Such differences in density should not be mistaken for thrombosis of the inferior cava (cf. **Figs. 21.1** and **138.1**).

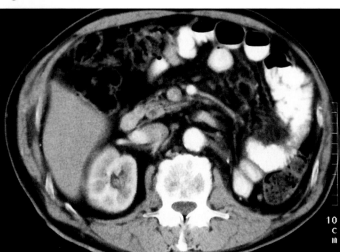

Fig. 20.2a

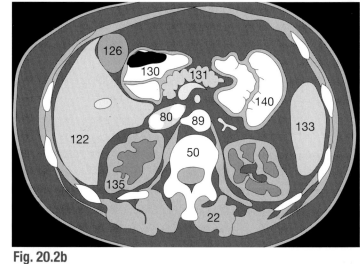

Fig. 20.2b

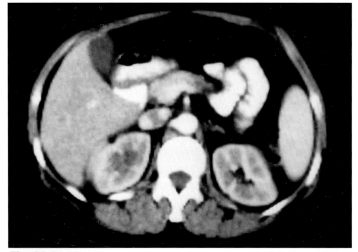

Fig. 20.3a

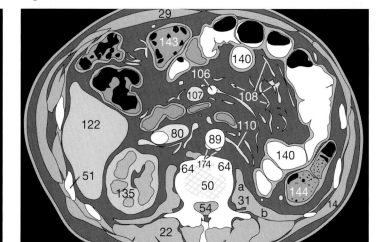

Fig. 20.3b

If we trace the inferior vena cava cranially toward the right atrium, additional flow phenomena become apparent as more veins empty into it. The cava has spiraling eddies of inhomogeneous density (➡ in **Fig. 21.1**) caused by mixing of the blood as described on the previous page. Moments later such inhomogeneities are no longer evident in the lumen **(80)** and density levels are identical to those in the aorta **(89)** (**Fig. 21.2a, b**).

By the way, did you notice the artherosclerotic plaque in the dorsal wall of the aorta (**174** in **89** in **Fig. 20.3a**)? This plaque appears also in **Figure 21.2a**. The patient had well-developed osteophytes **(64)** on the vertebral bodies **(50)**.

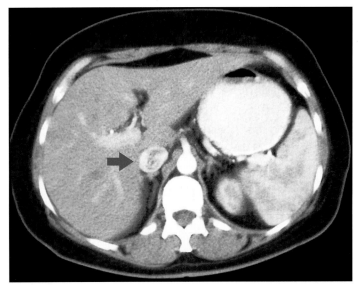

Fig. 21.1

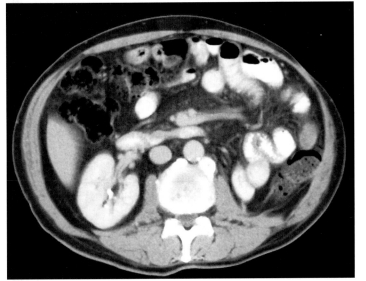

Fig. 21.2a

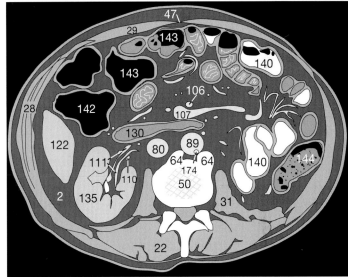

Fig. 21.2b

Details Specific for Spiral CT

If data acquisition begins immediately after CM has been administered, the concentration of CM in the axillary, subclavian, and brachiocephalic **(91)** veins might be high enough to cause major artifacts **(3)** in the thoracic inlet. In images such as in **Figure 21.3**, it is not possible to assess the lung or neighboring axillary tissues.

An SCT of the thorax should therefore be obtained from caudal to cranial. In that way structures near the diaphragm are imaged first and when cranial parts are scanned the CM will have been spread after having passed the pulmonary circulation. This trick helps avoid the artifacts **(3)** shown in **Figure 21.3**.

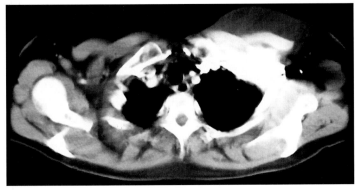

Fig. 21.3a

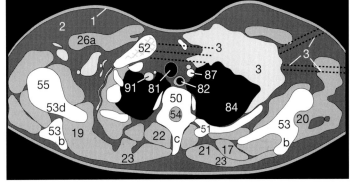

Fig. 21.3b

Adverse Reactions to Contrast Media

Adverse reactions are rare; most appear during the first 30 minutes, 70% of cases occur within the first 5 minutes after CM injection [13]. Only high-risk patients need to be supervised for more than 30 minutes. Since such patients can usually be recognized by taking a thorough medical history, they can be premedicated accordingly (see p. 14).

If, despite precautions, erythema develops after an i.v. injection of CM, perhaps also hives, itching, nausea or vomiting, or in extreme cases even hypotension or circulatory shock or shortness of breath, the countermeasures listed below must be initiated immediately. Remember that i.v. injection of H_1- and H_2-receptor antagonists does not alleviate symptoms immediately. There is a period of latency, and these antagonists are therefore primarily effective in preventing the symptoms from worsening and spreading. Serious incidents (pulmonary edema, circulatory shock, convulsions) occur very rarely with the new contrast media; they require immediate intensive care.

Be sure to document any incident in your report. Radiologists performing future examinations will be forewarned about the patient's sensitivity to CM.

Therapy of Adverse Reactions

▶ Gastrointestinal complications
(nausea and vomiting)

- Place the patient in lateral decubitus position to avoid aspiration
- H_1-receptor antagonist with good anti-emetic action (e.g., prochlorperazine, 5–10 mg, i.v.)
- H_1-receptor antagonist with potent anti-allergic effect (e.g., diphenhydramine, 25–50 mg) slowly i.v., **not to be mixed with:**
- H_2-receptor antagonist (e.g., cimetidine, 300 mg)
- if necessary, oxygen through nasal prongs (2–3 l/min)

▶ Reactions of skin and mucous membranes
(erythema, pruritis, hives, edema)

- Glucocorticoids i.v. (e.g., methylprednisolone 100–250 mg)
- H_1-receptor antagonist (e.g., prochlorperazine, 5–10 mg) slowly i.v., **not to be mixed with:**
- H_2-receptor antagonist (e.g., cimetidine, 300 mg)

only in extreme cases also:

- Adrenaline (0.1–0.3 mg, s.c.)

▶ Respiratory complications (dyspnea, asthma)
(stridor, bronchial spasms, laryngeal edema)

- Patient must sit up! (semi-upright position)
- Bronchodilator, aerosol (e.g., 1–2 inhalations)
- Oxygen through nasal prongs (2–3 l/min)

only in extreme cases also:

- Theophylline, slowly i.v. (e.g., 5 mg/kg bw) watch for tachycardial arrhythmia!
- Glucocorticoids i.v. (e.g., methylprednisolone 100–250 mg)
- Emergency intubation or in cases of laryngeal edema, cricoid puncture and intensive care

▶ Cardiovascular complications
(drop in blood pressure accompanied by bradycardia)

- Patient must lie flat, legs elevated
- Volume substitution (e.g., 500–1000 ml Ringer's solution)
- Atropine i.v. (e.g. 0.5–1.0 mg) repeated, if necessary up to 3.0 mg

only in extreme cases also:

- Oxygen through nasal prongs (2–3 l/min)
- Dopamine i.v. (e.g., 5–10 µg/kg bw/min)
- Monitoring: ECG and blood pressure!

▶ Anaphylactic shock
(extreme hypotension and tachycardia)

- Immediately call anesthesiologist or activate cardiac arrest team!
- Patient in supine position, legs elevated!
- Rapid volume substitution with colloidal substitute (e.g., dextran solution, no hypotonic solution!)
- Adrenaline (0.1–1.0 mg as 1–10 ml of 1:10 000 dilution = 0.1 mg/ml) slowly i.v. Special monitoring of patients with history of cardiovascular problems
- Oxygen through nasal prongs (2–3 l/min)
- ECG and blood pressure monitoring
  if hypotension persists:
- Dopamine i.v. (e.g., 5–10 µg/kg bw/min) H_1-receptor antagonist (e.g., prochlorperazine, 5–10 mg)
- slowly i.v., **not to be mixed with:** H_2-receptor antagonist (e.g., cimetidine, 300 mg)
- Artificial respiration, if necessary
- Intensive care unit

Thyrotoxic Crisis

Fortunately, these incidents are very rare with nonionized contrast media. Nevertheless, the uptake of iodine by the thyroid gland should be blocked before i.v. application of CM by administering a thyrostatic drug such as sodium perchlorate (Irenat) if the patient has a medical history of hyperthyroidism. As an alternative, the synthesis of monoiodotyrosin and diiodotyrosin can be blocked by carbimazole, for example. Both treatments take approximately 1 week to become fully effective. Effectiveness must be determined by repeating the thyroid function tests (see **Table 14.1**).

In cases with latent thyroid function, the use of iodine containing CM can elicit clinical hyperthyroidism or even a thyroid crisis. The symptoms may include diarrhea, muscle weakness, and paralysis as well as fever, sweating, dehydration, fear and restlessness, or even tachycardia/tachyarrhythmia. The main problem is the long period of latency before the thyrotoxic crisis becomes manifest.

Therapy

▶ **of thyrotoxic crisis**

- Always intensive care
- Thiamazol 150–200 mg/d i.v.
- Electrolyte substitution (3–4 l/d)
- Calorie substitution (3000 kcal/d)
- Cooling of the body
- Beta-blocker (special monitoring of cardiac patients)
- Thrombosis prophylaxis
- In extreme cases: plasmapheresis
- If needed: sedatives

Cranial CT examinations (CCT) can often be performed without having to give CM. In cases of sudden neurological deficits, for example when it is necessary to determine whether there is intracranial hemorrhage or infarction, no CM need be used. Intracranial metastases or tumors, however, can be more easily detected in contrast-enhanced images because the BBB surrounding the lesion is abnormal. This also holds true for the staging of brain infarctions or for localizing inflammatory foci.

Selection of the Image Plane

First a sagittal planning topogram (scanogram) is acquired at low resolution. This image serves to determine the desired scan angle and planes **(Fig. 24.1)**. The orbitomeatal line is usually selected because its fixed points are readily defined: the top of the orbit and the external auditory meatus. Although there are a number of alternatives, this plane is simple to repeat in follow-up examinations, making comparisons more reliable. Most radiologists scan the posterior fossa in thinner, closer slices (2/4 = 2-mm slice and 4-mm feed) than the supratentorial planes (8/8) in order to minimize artifacts due to the beam-hardening effect of the temporal bones.

When printing the hard copy, the correct orientation is important: most radiologists print the images so that they are seen from caudal. The hemispheres appear laterally reversed on the film. Only few departments of neurosurgery make exceptions: they prefer the cranial view because it usually corresponds to that seen by the surgical team.

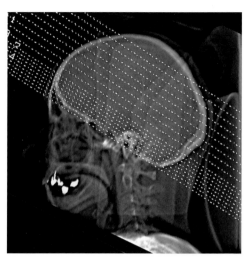

Fig. 24.1

A Systematic Sequence for Reading Cranial CT Images

Each radiologist is free to develop his or her own approach to reading the images. There is no "one and only" strategy. It is, however, useful to keep to a good sequence once it has been established. It helps avoid overlooking even small lesions. The checklist proposed below is one possible systematic order for image interpretation which has proven to be a good guideline for beginners in our courses. When analyzing the images you should always consider the age of the patient. The aging brain shows enlarged CSF spaces due to physiologic brain involution (see p.48). If you suspect the presence of a focal lesion, first check the neighboring scans, both above and below, in order to avoid misinterpreting simple partial volume effects **(Fig. 27.1a)**.

Since hard copies of cranial bone windows are expensive, they are not often printed and radiologists must examine this window on the monitor for pathologic changes, e.g. destructive bone lesions or fractures.

The following pages will give you a survey of normal cranial anatomy. Variations from the norm and pathologic changes are dealt with on pages 48 to 61. The number codes for the drawings are in the front foldout.

Checklist for Reading Cranial CTs
➡ Age of the patient? Medical history?
➡ Posttraumatic changes in the soft-tissue structures: bruises/tumors?
➡ Normal contours of quadrigeminal and basal cisterns? (Risk of brainstem herniation)
➡ Size and contours of ventricles and SAS appropriate to patient's age?
➡ Any blockage to flow of CSF (obstructive hydrocephalus) or signs of brain edema (=effaced sulci)?
➡ Asymmetries: due to head position or true asymmetry?
➡ Plain or contrast-enhanced CT: cerebral arteries regular? (Especially after injection of CM)
➡ Calcifications in the choroid plexus and pineal body only? (Common findings.) Any additional hyperdense foci?
➡ Paraventricular white matter and cortex inconspicuous and well defined? Any focal lesions or local edema?
➡ Basal ganglia and internal capsule intact? (Most common locations of cerebral infarctions)
➡ Brainstem, pons, and cerebellum normal?
➡ Skull checked for fractures and metastases in the bone window?

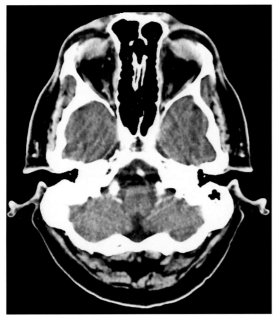

Fig. 25.1a

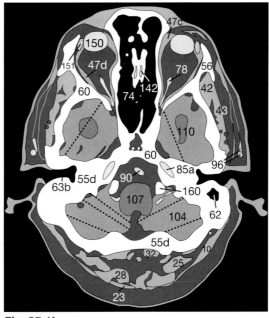

Fig. 25.1b

The scan usually begins at the base of the skull and continues upward. Since the hard copies are oriented such that the sections are viewed from caudal, all structures appear as if they were left/right reversed (see p. 10). The small topogram shows you the corresponding position of each image.

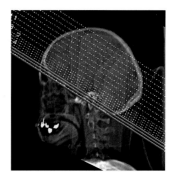

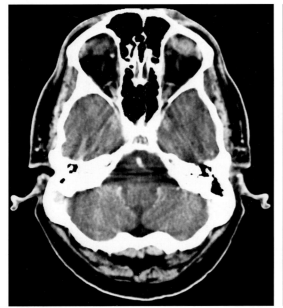

Fig. 25.2a

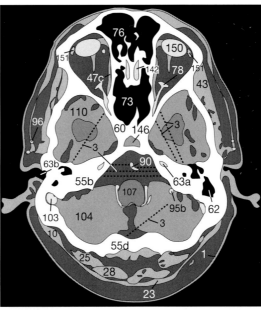

Fig. 25.2b

You should first check for any swellings in the soft tissues which may indicate trauma to the head. Always examine the condition of the basilar artery **(90)** in scans close to the base of the skull and the brainstem **(107)**. The view is often limited by streaks of artifacts **(3)** radiating from the temporal bones **(55b)**.

When examining trauma patients, remember to use the bone window to inspect the sphenoid bone **(60)**, the zygomatic bone **(56)**, and the calvaria **(55)** for fractures. In the caudal slices you can recognize basal parts of the temporal lobe **(110)** and the cerebellum **(104)**.

Orbital structures are usually viewed in another scanning plane (see pp. 31–38). In **Figure 25** we see only a partial slice of the upper parts of the globe **(150)**, the extraocular muscles **(47)**, and the olfactory bulb **(142)**.

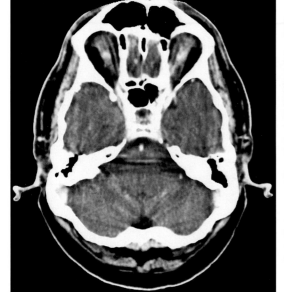

Fig. 25.3a

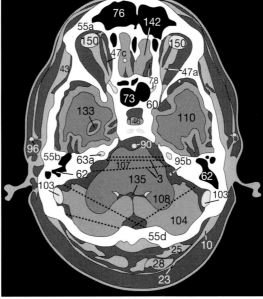

Fig. 25.3b

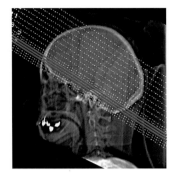

As the series of slices continues dorsally, the crista galli (162) and the basal parts of the frontal lobe (111) appear. The pons/medulla (107) are often obscured by artifacts (3). The pituitary gland (146) and stalk (147) are seen between the upper border of the sphenoid sinus (73) and the clinoid process (163). Of the dural sinuses, the sigmoid sinus (103) can be readily identified. The basilar artery (90) and the superior cerebellar artery (95a) lie anterior to the pons (107). The cerebellar tentorium (131), which lies dorsal to the middle cerebral artery (91b), shouldn't be mistaken for the posterior cerebral artery (91c) at the level depicted in **Figure 27.1a** on the next page. The inferior (temporal) horns of the lateral ventricles (133) as well as the 4th ventricle (135) can be identified in **Figure 26.3**. Fluid occurring in the normally air-filled mastoid cells (62) or in the frontal sinus (76) may indicate a fracture (blood) or an infection (effusion).

A small portion of the roof of the orbit (✶) can still be seen in **Figure 26.3**.

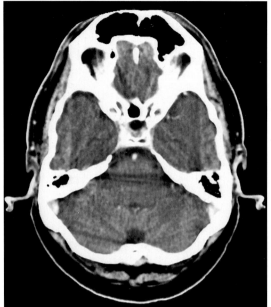

Fig. 26.1a

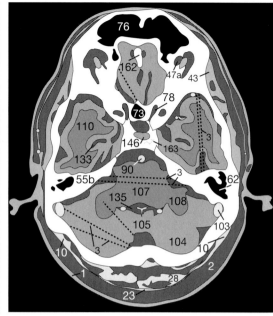

Fig. 26.1b

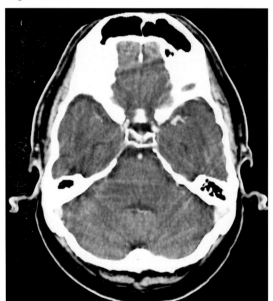

Fig. 26.2a

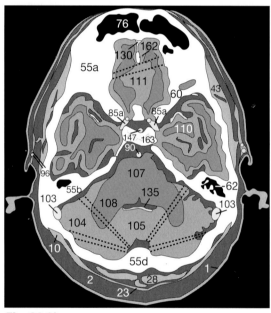

Fig. 26.2b

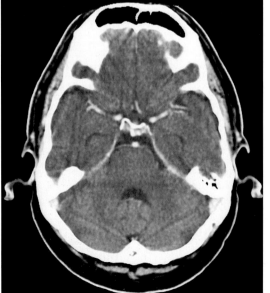

Fig. 26.3a

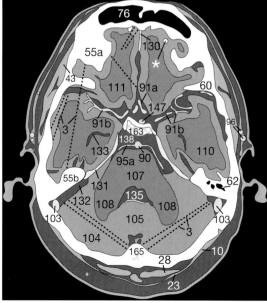

Fig. 26.3b

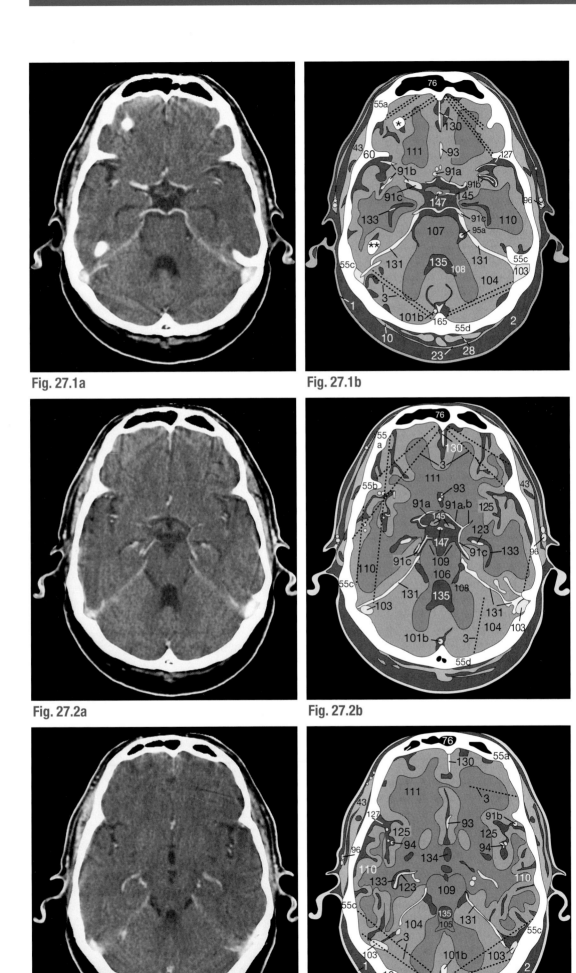

Fig. 27.1a

Fig. 27.1b

Fig. 27.2a

Fig. 27.2b

Fig. 27.3a

Fig. 27.3b

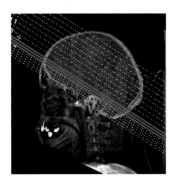

In **Figures 26.3a** and **27.1a** partial volume effects of the orbit (★) or the petrosal bone (★★) might also be misinterpreted as fresh hemorrhages in the frontal **(111)** or the temporal lobe **(110)**.

The cortex next to the frontal bone **(55a)** often appears hyperdense compared to adjacent brain parenchyma, but this is an artifact due to beam-hardening effects of bone. Note that the choroid plexus **(123)** in the lateral ventricle **(133)** is enhanced after i.v. infusion of CM. Even in plain scans it may appear hyperdense because of calcifications.

You will soon have recognized that the CCT images on these pages were taken after i.v. administration of CM: the vessels of the circle of Willis are markedly enhanced. The branches **(94)** of the middle cerebral artery **(91b)** are visible in the Sylvian fissure **(127)**. Even the pericallosal artery **(93)**, a continuation of the anterior cerebral artery **(91a)**, can be clearly identified. Nevertheless, it is often difficult to distinguish between the optic chiasm **(145)** and the pituitary stalk **(147)** because these structures have similar densities.

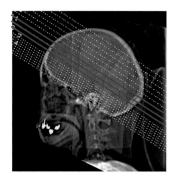

In addition to the above-mentioned cerebral arteries (93, 94), the falx cerebri (130) is a hyperdense structure. In Figure 28.2a you can see the extension of the hyperdense choroid plexus (123) through the foramen of Monro, which connects the lateral ventricles (133) with the 3rd ventricle (134). Check whether the contours of the lateral ventricles are symmetric.

A midline shift could be an indirect sign of edema. Calcifications in the pineal (148) are a common finding in adults, and are generally without any pathologic significance. Due to partial volume effects, the upper parts of the tentorium (131) often appear without clear margins so that it becomes difficult to demarcate the cerebellar vermis (105) and hemispheres (104) from the occipital lobe (112). It is particularly important to carefully inspect the internal capsule (121) and the basal ganglia: caudate nucleus (117), putamen (118), and globus pallidus (119) as well as the thalamus (120). Consult the number codes in the front foldout for the other structures not specifically mentioned on these pages.

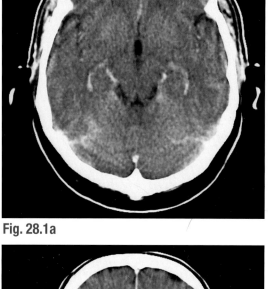

Fig. 28.1a

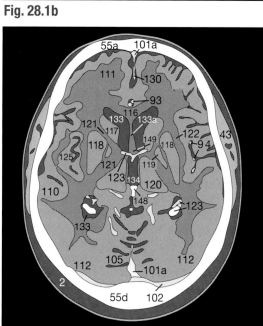

Fig. 28.1b

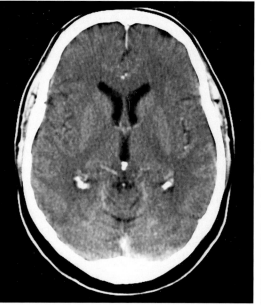

Fig. 28.2a

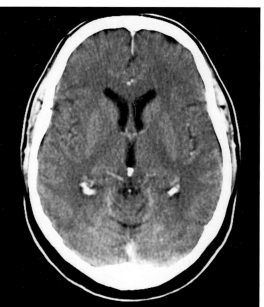

Fig. 28.2b

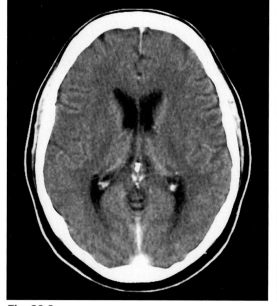

Fig. 28.3a

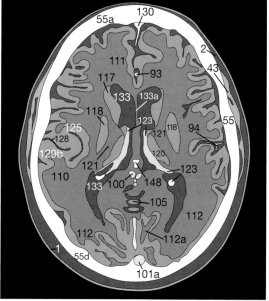

Fig. 28.3b

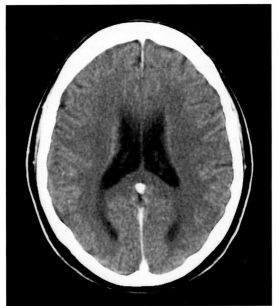

Fig. 29.1a

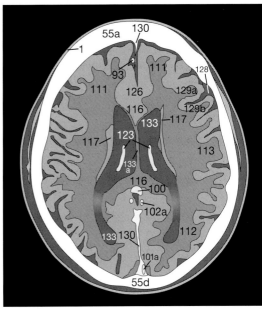

Fig. 29.1b

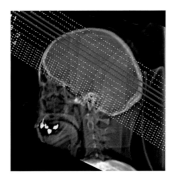

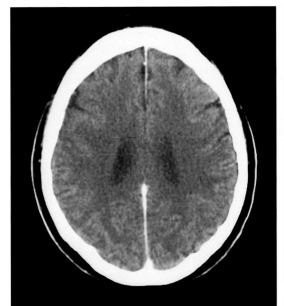

Fig. 29.2a

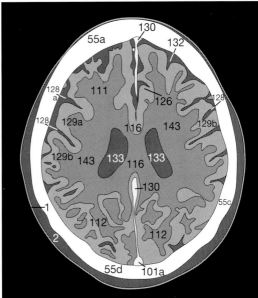

Fig. 29.2b

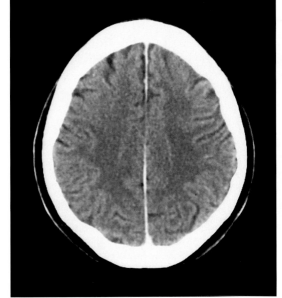

Fig. 29.3a

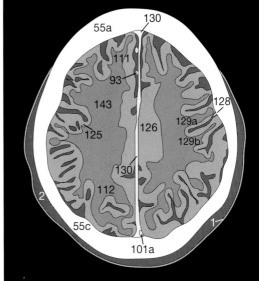

Fig. 29.3b

The position of the patient's head is not always as straight as in our example. Even small inclinations may lead to remarkably asymmetric pictures of the ventricular system, though in reality it is perfectly normal. You may see only a partial slice of the convex contours of the lateral ventricles **(133)**. This could give you the impression that they are not well defined **(Fig. 29.1a)**. The phenomenon must not be confused with brain edema: as long as the sulci (external SAS) are not effaced, but configured regularly, the presence of edema is rather improbable. For evaluating the width of the SAS, the patient's age is an important factor. Compare the images on pages 48 and 50 in this context. The paraventricular and supraventricular white matter **(143)** must be checked for poorly circumscribed hypodense regions of edema due to cerebral infarction. As residues of older infarctions, cystic lesions may develop. In late stages they are well defined and show the same density as CSF (see p. 56).

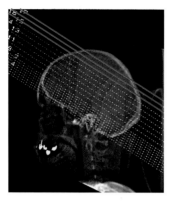

In the upper sections **(Figs. 30.1–30.3)** calcifications in the cerebral falx **(130)** often appear. You should differentiate this kind of lesion, which has no clinical significance, from calcified meningioma. The presence of CSF-filled sulci **(132)** in adults is an important finding with which to exclude brain edema. After a thorough evaluation of the cerebral soft-tissue window, a careful inspection of the bone window should follow. Continue to check for bone metastases or fracture lines. Only now is your evaluation of a cranial CT really complete.

Test yourself! Exercise 1:

Note from memory a systematic order for the evaluation of cranial CTs. If you have difficulties, return to the checklist on page 24.

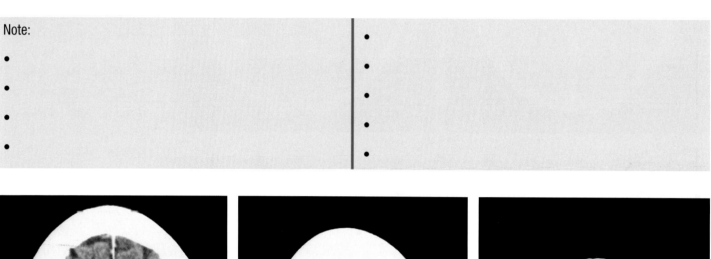

Note:

-
-
-
-

-
-
-
-
-

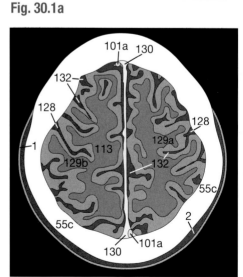

Fig. 30.1a

Fig. 30.2a

Fig. 30.3a

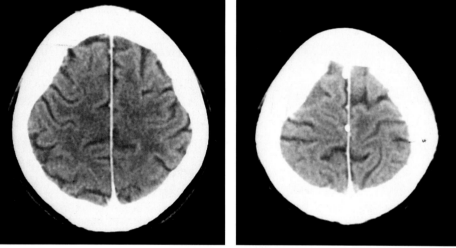

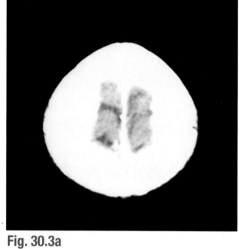

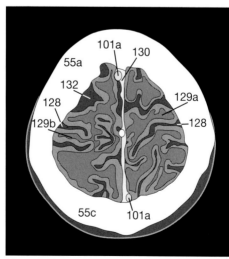

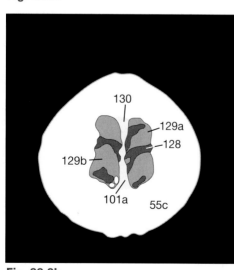

Fig. 30.1b

Fig. 30.2b

Fig. 30.3b

On the following pages the atlas of normal anatomy continues with scans of the orbits (axial), the face (coronal), and the petrosal bones (axial and coronal). After these you will find the most common anatomic variations, typical phenomena caused by partial volume effects and the most important intracranial pathologic changes on pages 48 to 58.

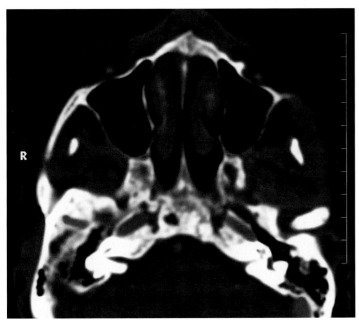

Fig. 31.1a

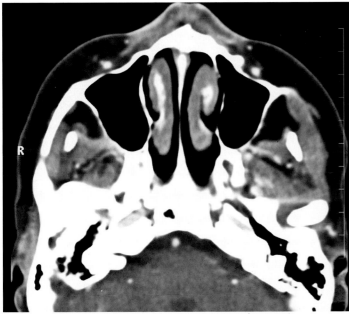

Fig. 31.1b

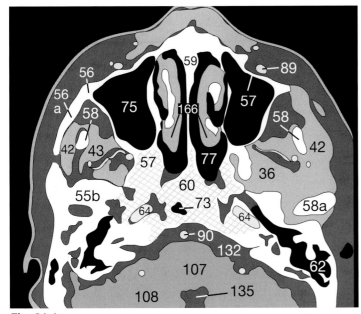

Fig. 31.1c

The face and the orbits are usually studied in thin slices (2 mm) using 2-mm collimation steps. The orientation of the scanning plane is comparable to that for CCTs (see p. 24). In the sagittal topogram the line of reference lies parallel to the floor of the orbit at an angle of about 15° to horizontal (Fig. 31.2).

The printouts are usually presented in the view from caudal: all structures on the right side of the body appear on the left, and vice versa.

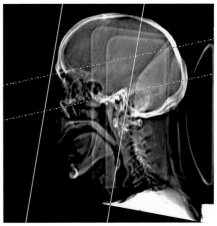

Fig. 31.2

Alterations in the soft structures of the orbits and the paranasal sinuses can be readily evaluated in the soft-tissue window (Fig. 31.1b). For the detection of a tumor-related arrosion of bone, or a fracture, the bone window should also be checked (Fig. 31.1a). The following pages therefore present each scan level in both windows. The accompanying drawing (Fig. 31.1c) refers to both. The number codes for all drawings are found in the legend in the front foldout.

On the lower slices of the orbits you will see parts of the maxillary sinus (75), the nasal cavity (77) with the conchae (166), the sphenoid sinus (73), and the mastoid cells (62) as air-filled spaces. If there is fluid or a soft-tissue mass this may indicate a fracture, an infection, or a tumor of the paranasal sinuses. For examples of such diseases, see pages 58 to 61.

Two parts of the mandible appear on the left side: in addition to the coronoid process (58), the temporomandibular joint with the head of the mandible (58a) is seen on the left. The carotid artery, however, is often difficult to discern in the carotid canal (64), whether in the soft-tissue or bone window.

In the petrous part of the temporal bone (55b), the tympanic cavity (66) and the vestibular system are visible. For a more detailed evaluation of the semicircular canals and the cochlea, images obtained with the petrous bone technique are more appropriate (pp. 44–47). CM was infused intravenously before the examination of the orbits. The branches of both the facial and angular vessels (89) as well as the basilar artery (90) therefore appear markedly hyperdense in the soft-tissue window (Fig. 31.1b).

It is not always possible to achieve a precise sagittal position of the head. Even a slight tilt **(Fig. 32.1)** will make the temporal lobe **(110)** appear on one side, whereas on the other side the mastoid cells **(62)** can be seen.

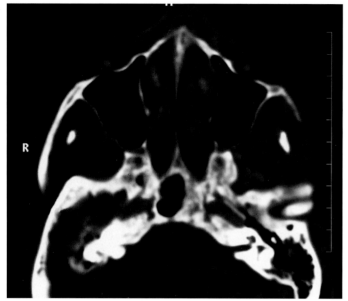

Fig. 32.1a

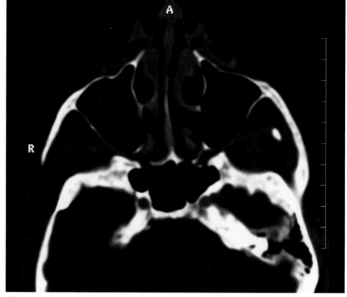

Fig. 32.2a

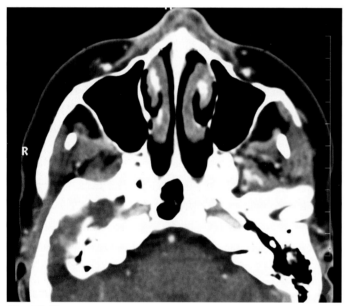

Fig. 32.1b

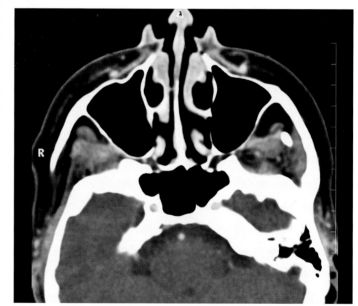

Fig. 32.2b

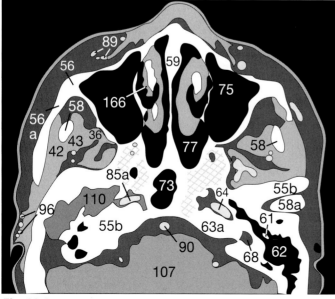

Fig. 32.1c

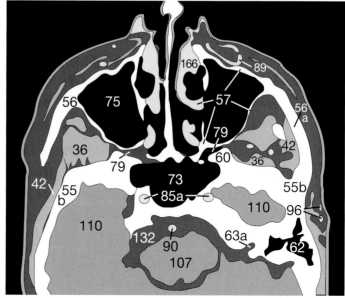

Fig. 32.2c

As experience shows, it is difficult to determine the course of the internal carotid artery **(85a)** through the base of the skull and to demarcate the pterygopalatine fossa **(79)**, through which, among other structures, the greater palatine nerve and the nasal branches of the pterygopalatine ganglion (from CN V and CN VII) pass.

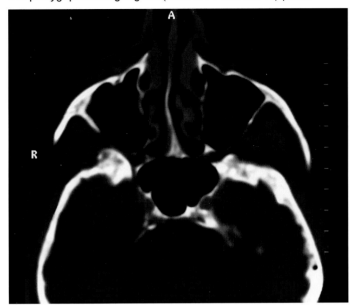

Fig. 33.1a

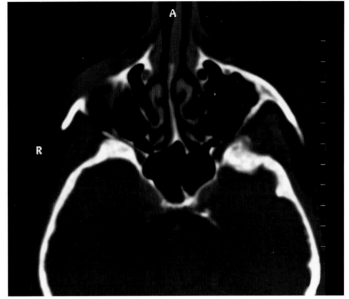

Fig. 33.2a

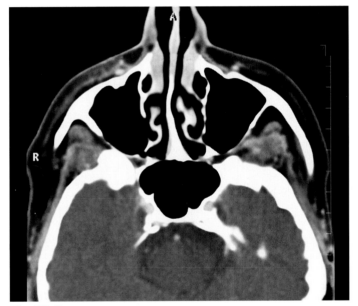

Fig. 33.1b

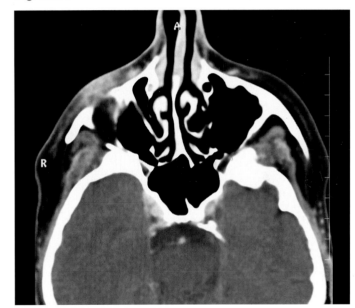

Fig. 33.2b

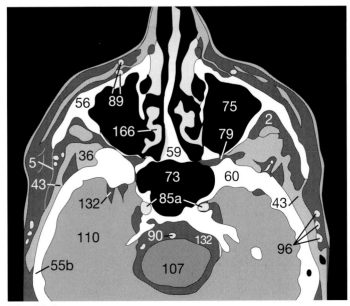

Fig. 33.1c

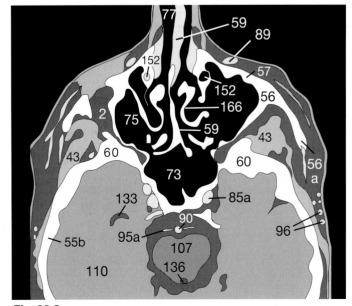

Fig. 33.2c

On the floor of the orbit, the short inferior oblique muscle **(47f)** often seems poorly delineated from the lower lid. This is due to the similar densities of these structures. Directly in front of the clinoid process/dorsum sellae **(163)** lies the pituitary gland **(146)** in its fossa, which is laterally bordered by the carotid siphon **(85a)**.

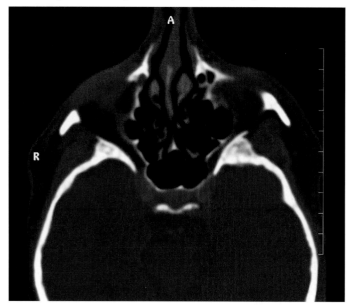

Fig. 34.1a

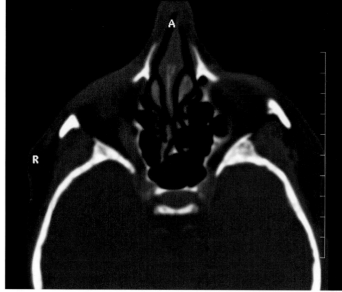

Fig. 34.2a

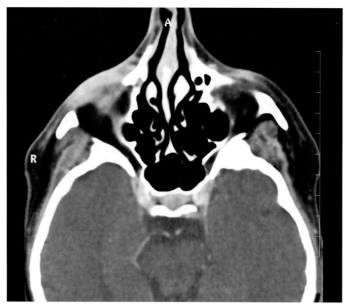

Fig. 34.1b

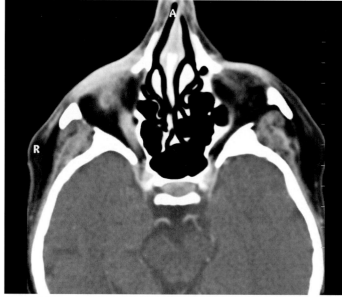

Fig. 34.2b

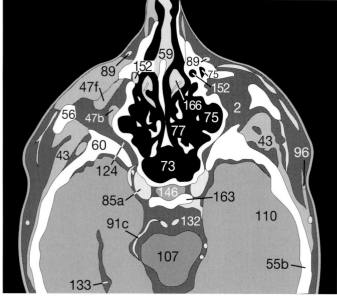

Fig. 34.1c

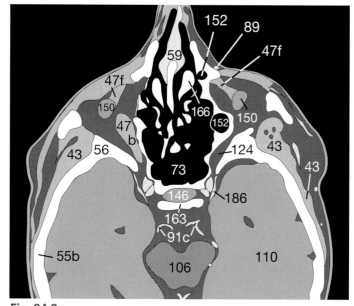

Fig. 34.2c

Small inclinations of the head cause slightly asymmetric views of the globe (150) and the extraocular muscles (47). The medial wall of the nasolacrimal duct (152) is often so thin that it cannot be differentiated. At first sight the appearance of the clinoid process (163), between the pituitary stalk (147) and the carotid siphon (85a) on the left side only, may be confusing in **Figure 35.2b**.

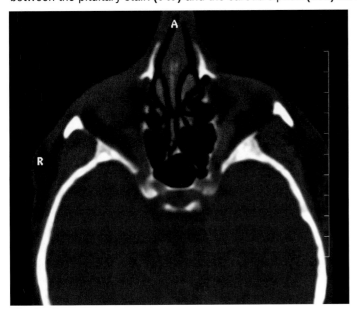

Fig. 35.1a

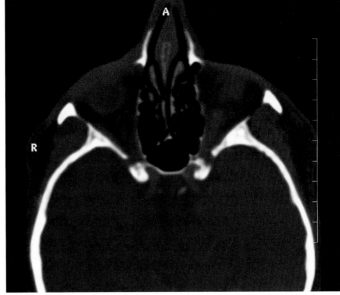

Fig. 35.2a

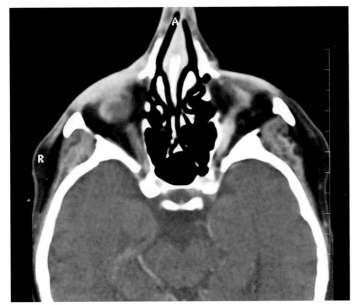

Fig. 35.1b

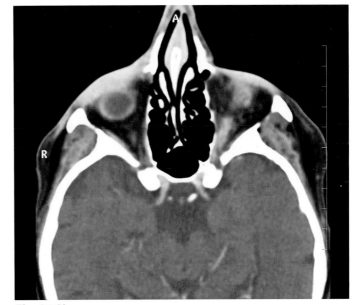

Fig. 35.2b

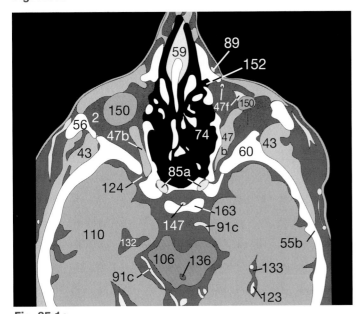

Fig. 35.1c

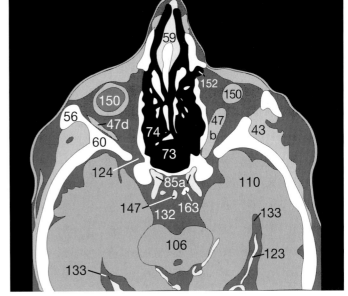

Fig. 35.2c

After intravenous injection of CM, the branches of the middle cerebral artery (91b) originating from the internal carotid artery (85a), are readily distinguished. The gray shade of the optic nerves (78) as they pass through the chiasm (145) to the optic tracts (144) however, is very similar to that of the surrounding CSF (132). You should always check on the symmetry of the extraocular muscles (47) in the retrobulbar fatty tissue (2).

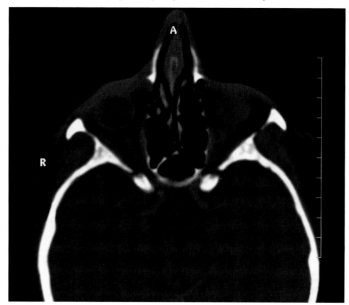

Fig. 36.1a

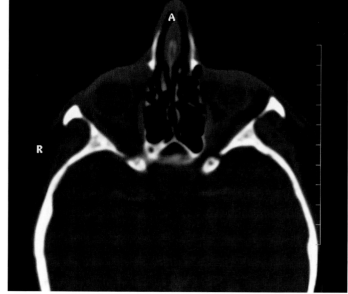

Fig. 36.2a

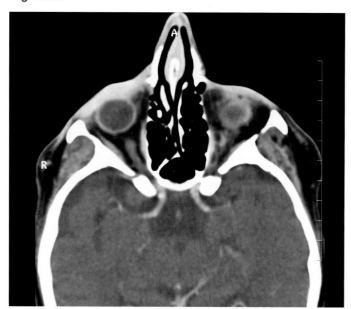

Fig. 36.1b

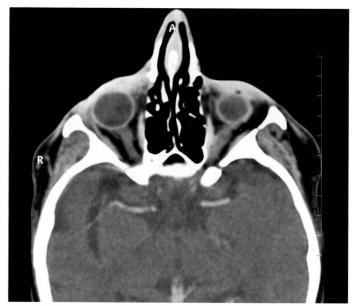

Fig. 36.2b

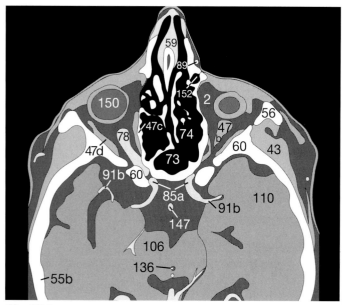

Fig. 36.1c

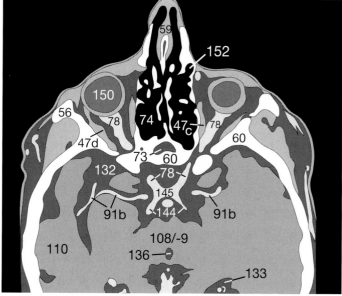

Fig. 36.2c

In the globe **(150)** you can now see the hyperdense lens **(150a)**. Notice the oblique course of the ophthalmic artery **(★)** crossing the optic nerve **(78)** in the retrobulbar fatty tissue **(2)**. **Figure 37.2b** shows a slight swelling **(7)** of the right lacrimal gland **(151)** compared to the left one (see **Fig. 38.1b**).

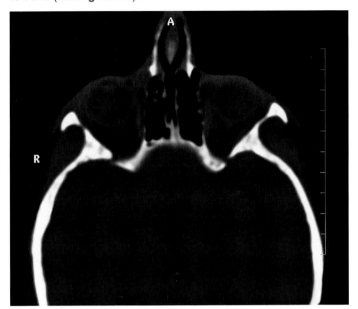

Fig. 37.1a

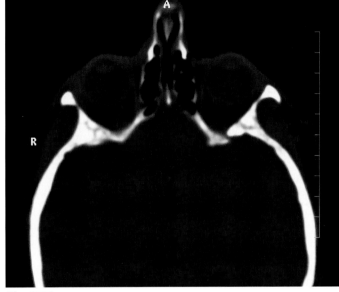

Fig. 37.2a

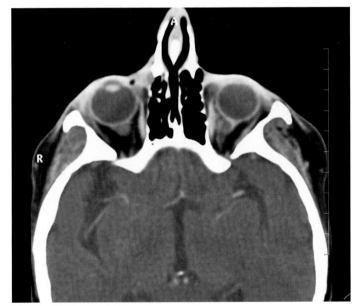

Fig. 37.1b

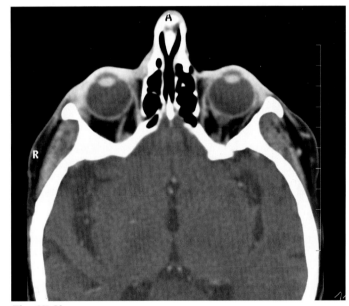

Fig. 37.2b

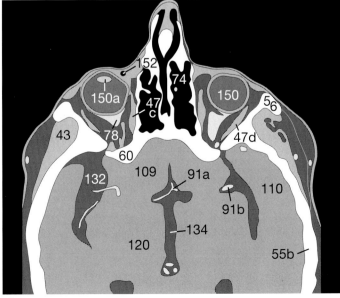

Fig. 37.1c

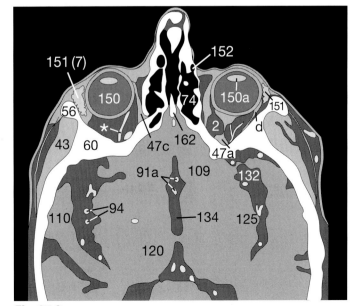

Fig. 37.2c

Figure 38.1b clarifies that in this case there is indeed an inflammation or tumor-like thickening **(7)** in the right lacrimal gland **(151)**. The superior rectus muscle **(47a)** appears at the roof of the orbit and immediately next to it lies the levator palpebrae muscle **(46)**. Due to similar densities, these muscles are not easily differentiated.

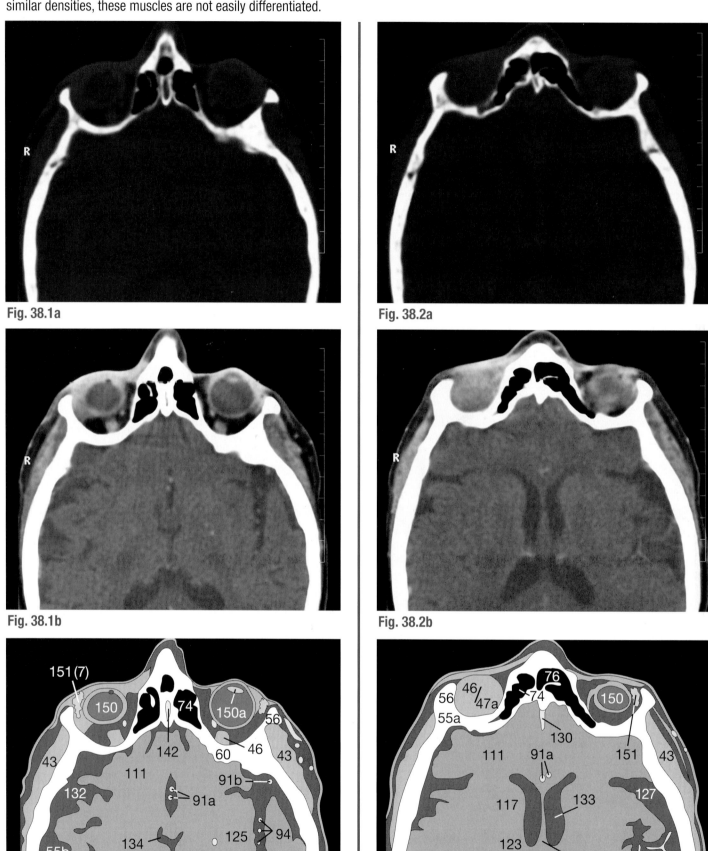

Fig. 38.1a

Fig. 38.2a

Fig. 38.1b

Fig. 38.2b

Fig. 38.1c

Fig. 38.2c

The axial views of the orbits and the face end here with the appearance of the frontal sinus **(76)**. Examples of pathologic changes of the orbits or fractures of facial bones are found on pages 59 to 61.

The possibilities of angling the CT gantry are limited. In order to acquire scans in the coronal plane, the patient must therefore be positioned as shown in the planning topogram to the right **(Fig. 39.1)**. The patient should be in a prone position, with the head completely extended. When examining trauma patients, any lesions of the bones or ligaments of the cervical spine must always be excluded by conventional radiography prior to CCT.

Images viewed from anterior: the anatomic structures on the patient's right side appear on the left in the images and conversely, as if the examiner were facing the patient.

When looking for fractures, images are usually acquired in the thin-slice mode (slice and collimation, each 2 mm) and viewed on bone windows. Even fine fracture lines can then be detected. A suspected fracture of the zygomatic arch may require additional scans in the axial plane (see p. 32). In **Figure 39.2a** the inferior alveolar canal (✱) in the mandible **(58)** and the foramen rotundum (✱✱) in the sphenoid bone **(60)** are clearly visible. As for the previous chapter, the code numbers for the drawings are explained in the legend in the front foldout.

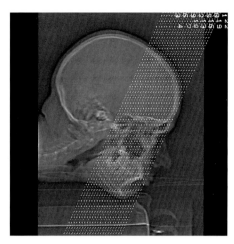

Abb. 39.1

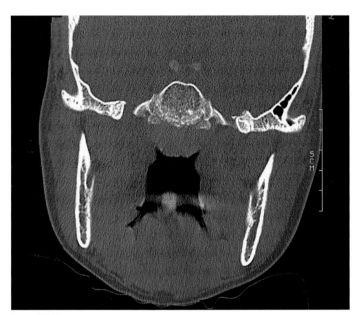

Fig. 39.2a

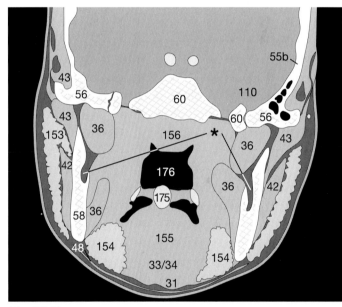

Fig. 39.2b

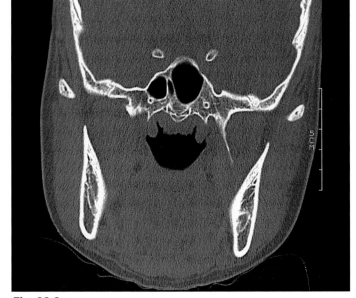

Fig. 39.3a

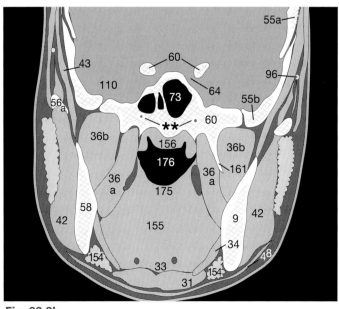

Fig. 39.3b

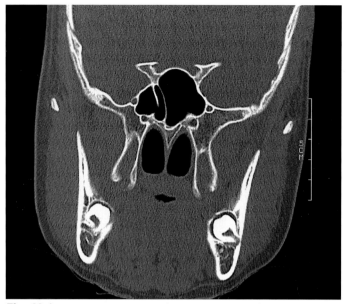

Fig. 40.1a

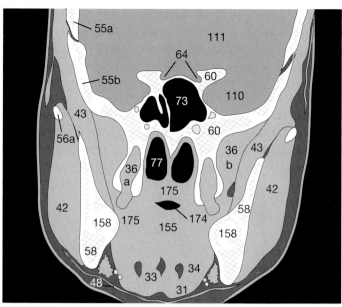

Fig. 40.1b

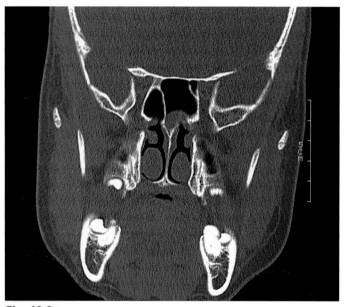

Fig. 40.2a

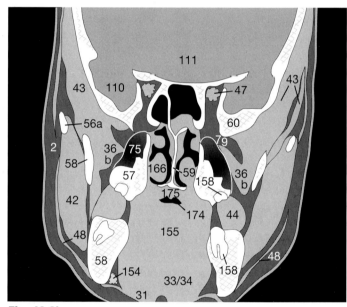

Fig. 40.2b

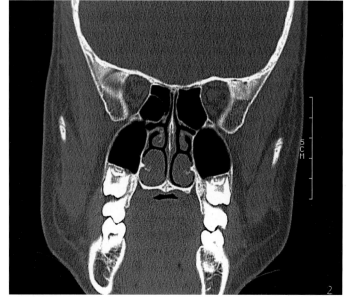

Fig. 40.3a

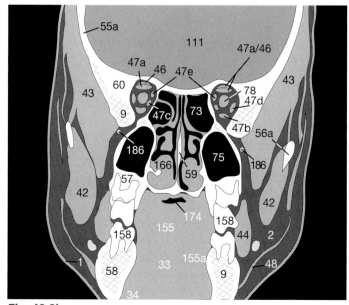

Fig. 40.3b

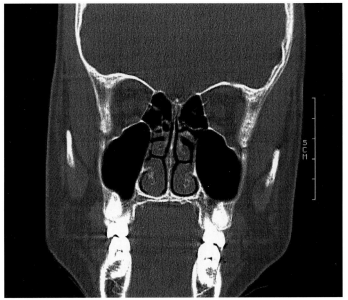

Fig. 41.1a

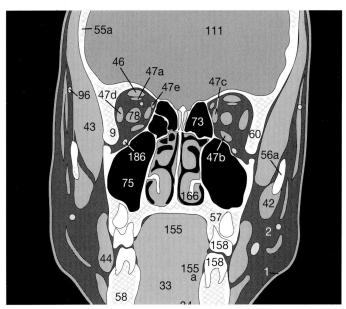

Fig. 41.1b

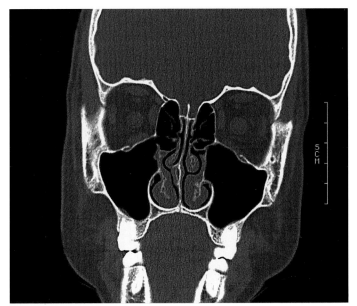

Fig. 41.2a

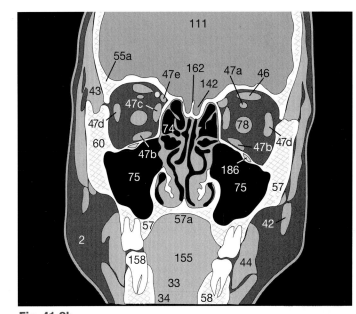

Fig. 41.2b

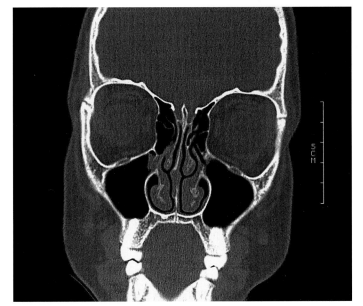

Fig. 41.3a

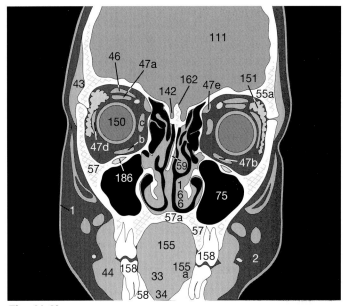

Fig. 41.3b

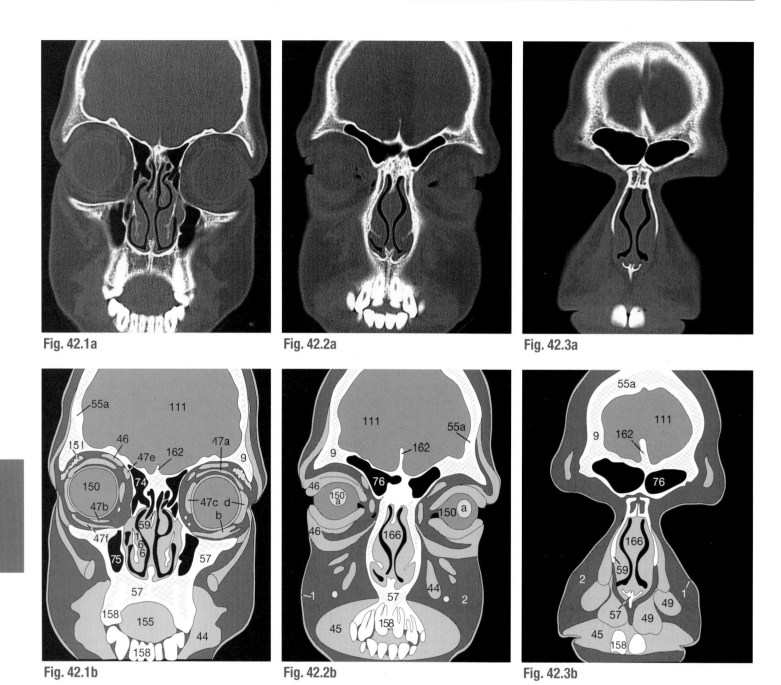

Fig. 42.1a

Fig. 42.2a

Fig. 42.3a

Fig. 42.1b

Fig. 42.2b

Fig. 42.3b

The insertions of the extraocular muscles on the globe **(150)** can also be clearly identified **(47 a–f)** in the anterior slices. The short inferior oblique muscle **(47f)**, however, is often seen only in coronal scanning planes, because it does not pass with the others muscles through the retrobulbar fatty connective tissue. The same problem occurs in axial scans of the face (compare **Figs. 34.2b** and **34.2c**). If a case of chronic sinusitis is suspected, it is very important to check whether the semilunar hiatus is open. It represents the main channel for discharging secretions of the paranasal sinuses. In **Figure 58.3** you will find examples of anatomic variations which narrow this channel and may promote chronic sinusitis.

Sometimes one discovers a congenitally reduced pneumatization of a frontal sinus **(76)** or an asymmetric arrangement of other paranasal sinuses without any pathologic consequences. You should always make sure that all paranasal sinuses are filled exclusively with air, that they are well defined and present no air-fluid levels. Hemorrhage into the paranasal sinuses or the detection of intracranial bubbles of air must be interpreted as an indirect sign of a fracture – you will find examples of such fractures on page 61.

On the previous pages you have learned about the normal anatomy of the brain, the orbits, and the face. It may be some time ago that you studied the technical basics of CT and about adequate preparation of the patient. Before going on with the anatomy of the temporal bone, it would be good to check on and refresh your knowledge of the last chapters. All exercises are numbered consecutively, beginning with the first one on page 30.

Without doubt, you will improve your understanding of the subject if you tackle the gaps in your knowledge instead of skipping problems or looking at the answers at the end of the book. Refer to the relevant pages only if you get stuck.

Exercise 2: Write down from memory the typical window parameters for images of the lungs, bones, and soft tissues. Note precisely the width and center of each window in HU and give reasons for the differences. If you have difficulties answering this question, go back to pages 12/13 to refresh your memory.

Lung/pleura window:	Center	Width	HU
Bone window:			
Soft-tissue window:			

Exercise 3: Which two types of oral CM do you know? What specific aspects must you consider when administering this kind of CM depending on the clinical problem? Are there any consequences for your list?

Oral CM (name)	Indication	Special schedule
●		
●		

Exercise 4: What aspects should you always clarify before referring your patients to a CT examination which probably requires the i.v. infusion of CM? The same applies if you consider referring someone to a venogram/angiogram or an IVU (both procedures are carried out with nonionic CM containing iodine). MRI examinations, however, are carried out with gadolinium as the CM. (The answers to questions 3 and 4 can be found on pp. 14 and 15.)

a)

b)

c)

Exercise 5: How would you differentiate between long structures such as vessels, nerves, or certain muscles and nodular structures such as lymph nodes or tumors? (You will find the answer on p. 11.)

Exercise 6: In which vessels might you find turbulence phenomena, caused by the CM injection, that must not be mistaken for a thrombus? (If you don't remember, check back to pp. 19–21.)

In order to evaluate the organ of hearing and balance, the petrosal bone is usually examined in thin slices without overlap (2/2). To ensure optimal resolution, the whole skull is not imaged, just the required part of the petrosal bone. The two petrosal bones **(55b)** are therefore enlarged and imaged separately. Only then is it possible to differentiate small structures like the ossicles **(61a–c)**, cochlea **(68)**, and the semicircular canals **(70a–c)**.

The topogram **(Fig. 44.1)** indicates the coronal imaging plane. The patient must be placed in a prone position with his or her head hyperextended. Note the pneumatization of the mastoid cells **(62)** and the usually thin walls of the outer auditory canal **(63b)**. Inflammation of these air-filled sinuses leads to characteristic effusion and swelling of the mucous membranes (see **Fig. 58.2a**).

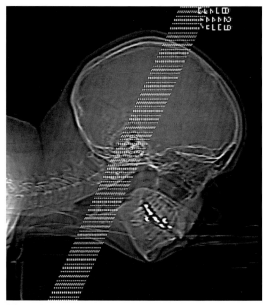

Fig. 44.1

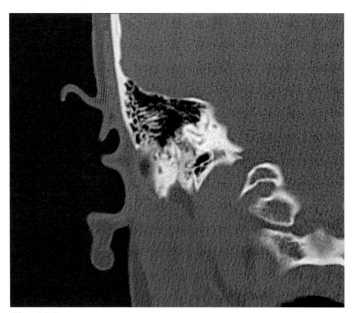

Fig. 44.2a

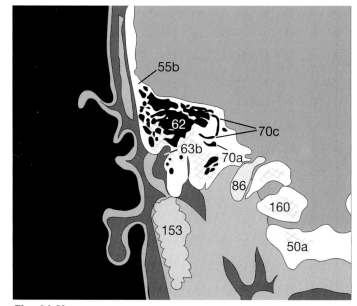

Fig. 44.2b

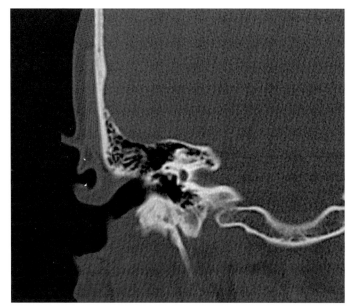

Fig. 44.3a

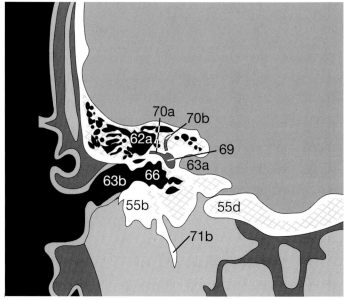

Fig. 44.3b

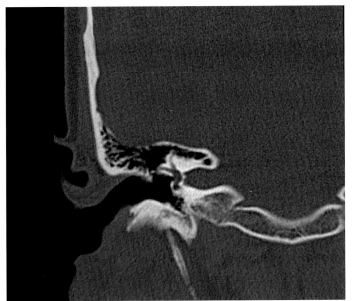

Fig. 45.1a

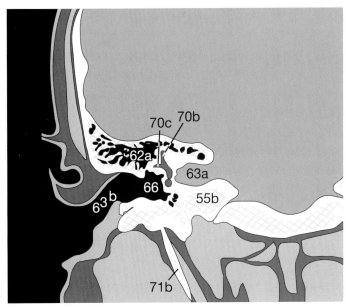

Fig. 45.1b

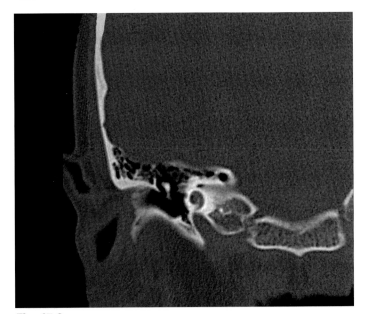

Fig. 45.2a

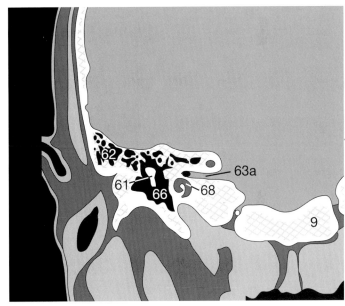

Fig. 45.2b

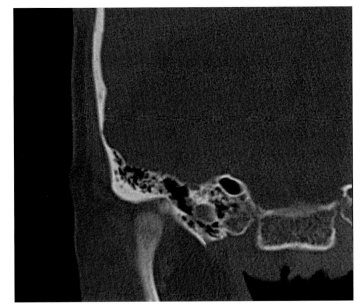

Fig. 45.3a

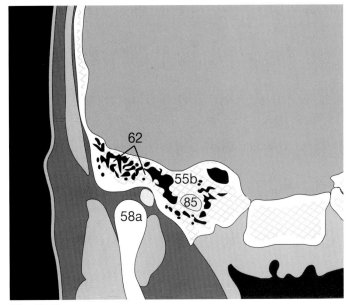

Fig. 45.3b

Analogous to coronal images, axial images are obtained with thin slices without overlap, i.e., 2 mm thickness and 2 mm increment and viewed on bone windows. The cerebellar hemispheres **(104)**, the temporal lobe **(110)**, and the soft tissues of the galea are therefore barely identifiable. Apart from the ossicles **(61a–c)** and the semicircular canals **(70a–c)**, the internal carotid artery **(64)**, the cochlea **(68)**, and the internal **(63a)** and external auditory canals **(63b)** are visualized. The funnel-shaped depression in the posterior rim of the petrosal bone **(Fig. 46.2a)** represents the opening of the perilymphatic duct (★★ = aqueduct of the cochlea) into the subarachnoid space. In **Figure 47.1a** note the localization of the geniculate ganglion of the facial nerve (★) ventral to the facial canal. The topogram **(Fig. 46.1a)** shows an axial plane of section, obtained with the patient lying supine.

Test Yourself!   Exercise No. 7:   Think about differential diagnoses involving effusion in the middle ear **(66)**, the outer auditory canal, or the mastoid cells **(62)** and compare your results with the cases shown on pages 58 and 60 to 61.

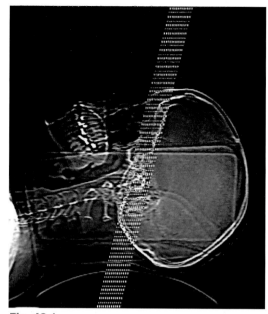

Fig. 46.1

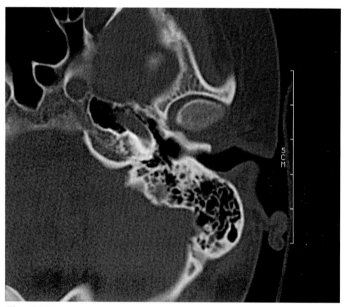

Fig. 46.2a

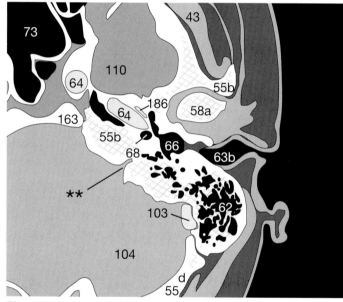

Fig. 46.2b

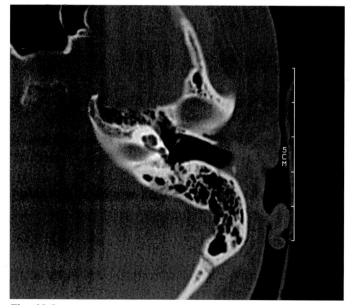

Fig. 46.3a

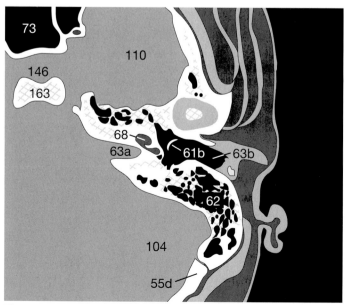

Fig. 46.3b

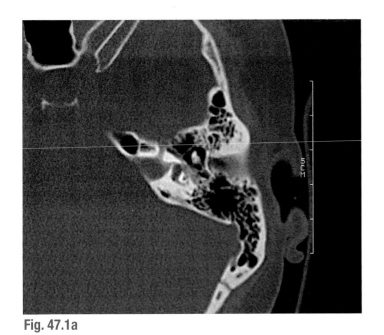

Fig. 47.1a

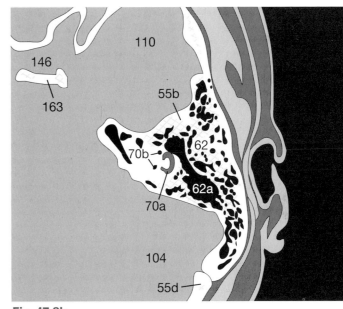

Fig. 47.1b

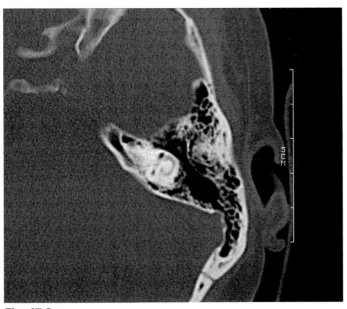

Fig. 47.2a

Fig. 47.2b

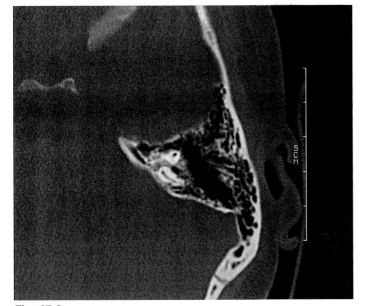

Fig. 47.3a

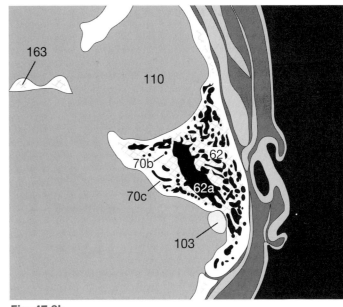

Fig. 47.3b

Do you remember the systematic sequence for evaluating CCT scans? If not, please go back to the checklist on page 24 or to your own notes on page 30.

After evaluating the soft tissues it is essential to examine the inner and outer CSF spaces. The width of the ventricles and the surface SAS increases continuously with age.

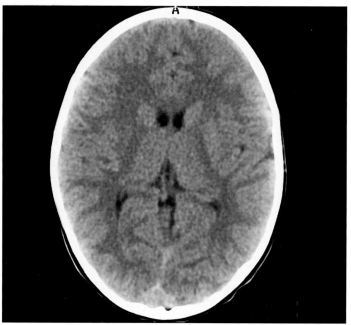

Fig. 48.1a

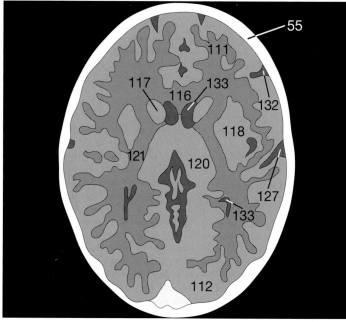

Fig. 48.1b

Since the brain of a child (Fig. 48.1a) fills the cranium (55), the outer subarachnoid space is scarcely visible, but with increasing age the sulci enlarge (Fig. 48.2a) and CSF (132) becomes visible between cortex and calvaria. In some patients this physiologic decrease in cortex volume is especially obvious in the frontal lobe (111). The space between it and the frontal bone (55a) becomes quite large. This so-called frontally emphasized brain involution should not be mistaken for pathologic atrophy of the brain or congenital microcephalus. If the CT scan in Figure 48.1a had been taken of an elderly patient, one would have to consider diffuse cerebral edema with pathologically effaced gyri. Before making a diagnosis of cerebral edema or brain atrophy you should therefore always check on the age of the patient.

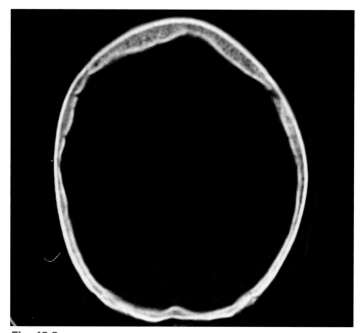

Fig. 48.2a

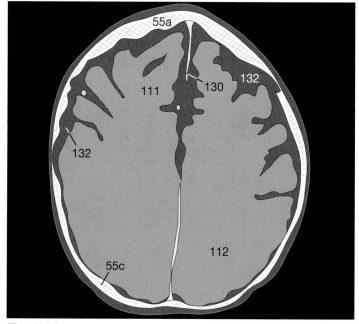

Fig. 48.2b

Figure 48.2a shows an additional variation from the norm. Especially in middle-aged female patients you will sometimes find hyperostosis of the frontal bone (55a) (Steward-Morel-Syndrome) without any pathologic significance. The frontal bone (55a) is internally thickened on both sides, sometimes with an undulating contour. In cases of doubt, the bone window can help to differentiate between normal spongiosa and malignant infiltration.

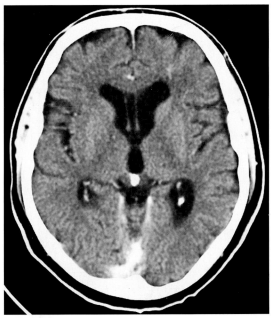

Fig. 49.1a

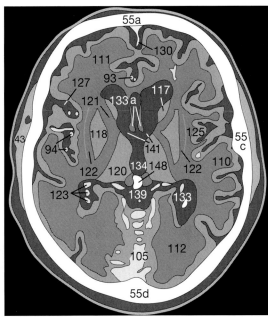

Fig. 49.1b

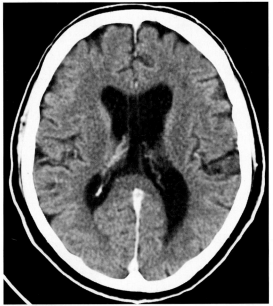

Fig. 49.2a

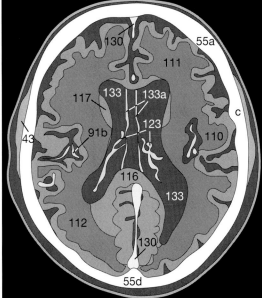

Fig. 49.2b

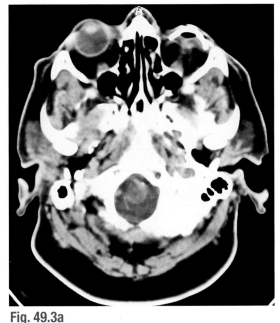

Fig. 49.3a

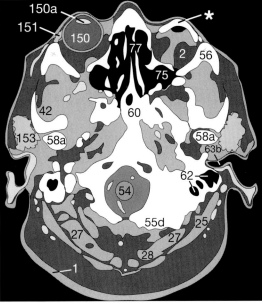

Fig. 49.3b

An incomplete fusion of the septum pellucidum (133a) can, as another variation, lead to the development of a so-called cavum of the septum pellucidum. Please review the normal scans in Figures 28.2a, 28.3a, and 29.1a for comparison. Usually only the part of the septum located between the two anterior horns of the lateral ventricles (Fig. 49.1a) is involved, less frequently the cavum extends all the way to the posterior horns (Fig. 49.2a).

In the plane of Figure 49.1, just medial of the head of the caudate nucleus (117), you can evaluate both foramina of Monro (141) which function as a route for the choroid plexus (123) and the CSF from the lateral ventricles (133) to the 3rd ventricle (134).

Refresh your anatomic skills by naming all other structures in Figure 49.1 and checking your results in the legend. The radiologist will rarely be confronted with an eye prosthesis (∗) after enucleation of a globe (150). In patients with a history of orbital tumor, a local relapse, i.e. in the retrobulbar space (2) has to be ruled out in check-up CT scans.

The CT scan of the orbit in Figure 49.3a showed minor postoperative change without any evidence of recurrent tumor.

One of the most important rules of CT scan interpretation is to always compare several adjacent planes (see pp. 10–11). If the head is tilted even slightly during the scan procedure, one lateral ventricle **(133)** for example, can appear in the image plane **(d_S)** whereas the contralateral ventricle is still outside the plane **(Fig. 50.1)**. Only its roof will appear. The computer therefore calculates a blurred, hypodense area which could be mistaken for a cerebral infarction **(Fig. 50.2a)**. By comparing this plane with the adjacent one below it **(Fig. 50.3a)** the situation becomes clear, since the asymmetric contours of the imaged ventricles are now obvious.

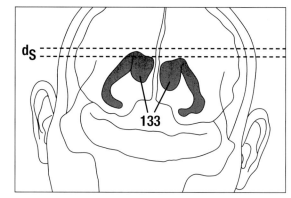

Fig. 50.1

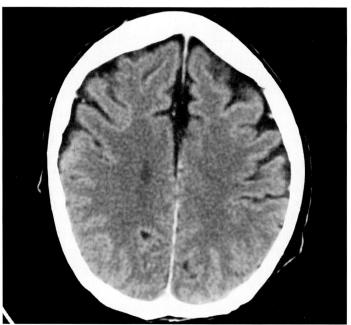

Fig. 50.2a

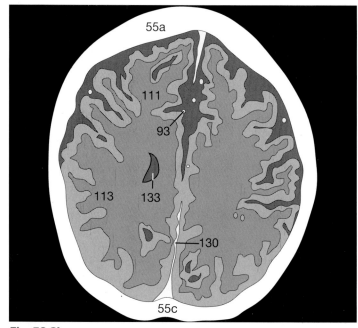

Fig. 50.2b

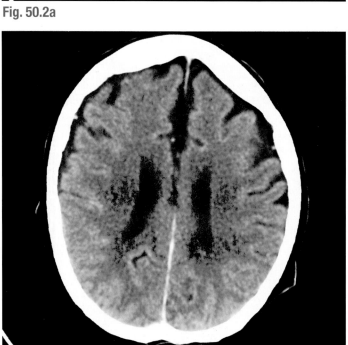

Fig. 50.3a

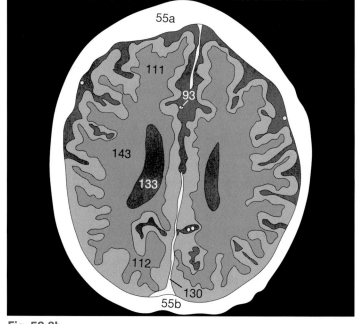

Fig. 50.3b

This example illustrates the importance of the correct placement of the patient's head. The exact position of the nose in an a.p. projection is obtained by using the gantry positioning lights. Involuntary movements of the head can be kept at a minimum by soft padding. In ventilated or unconscious patients an additional immobilization of the head with suitable bandings may be necessary.

One of the first steps in interpreting CCTs is the inspection of the soft tissues. Contusions with subcutaneous hematomas **(8)** may indicate skull trauma **(Fig. 50.1a)** and call for a careful search for an intracranial hematoma. Many injured patients cannot be expected to have their heads fixed for the duration of the CT scan, and this leads to considerable rotation. Asymmetric contours (★ in **Fig. 51.1a**) of the roof of the orbit **(55a)**, the sphenoid bone **(60)**, or the petrosal bone (not asymmetric in the illustrated examples!) are therefore frequent occurrences and may lead to misinterpretations of the hyperdense bone as a fresh intracranial hematoma.

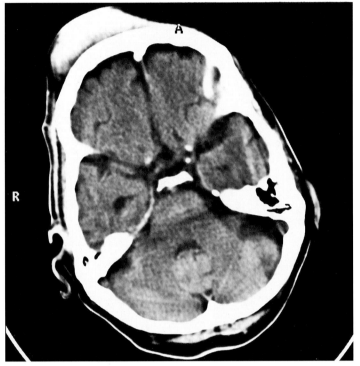

Fig. 51.1a

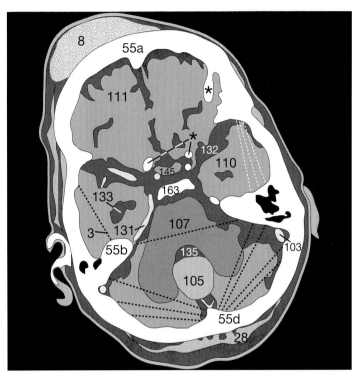

Fig. 51.1b

The question of whether it is just an asymmetric projection of the skull base or a real hematoma can be answered by comparing adjacent sections **(Fig. 51.2a)**. In this example the bones of the skull base caused the hyperdense partial volume effect. Despite the obvious right frontal extracranial contusion, intracranial bleeding could not be confirmed. Please note the considerable beam hardening (bone) artifacts **(3)** overlapping the brain stem **(107)**. Such artifacts would not appear in MR images of these levels.

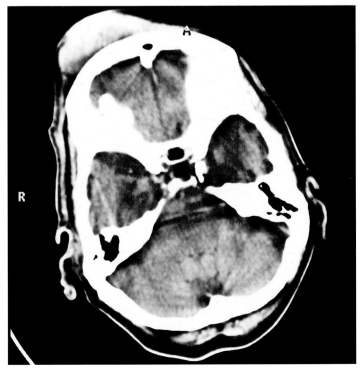

Fig. 51.2a

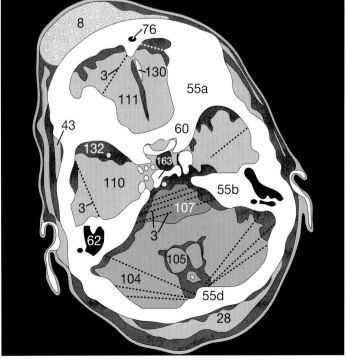

Fig. 51.2b

After having discussed that partial volume effects due to asymmetric projections (i.e., **55b** in **Fig. 52.2b**) may be misinterpreted as acute hematomas, this chapter will point out the characteristics of the different types of intracranial hemorrhage.

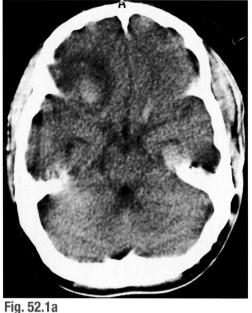

Fig. 52.1a

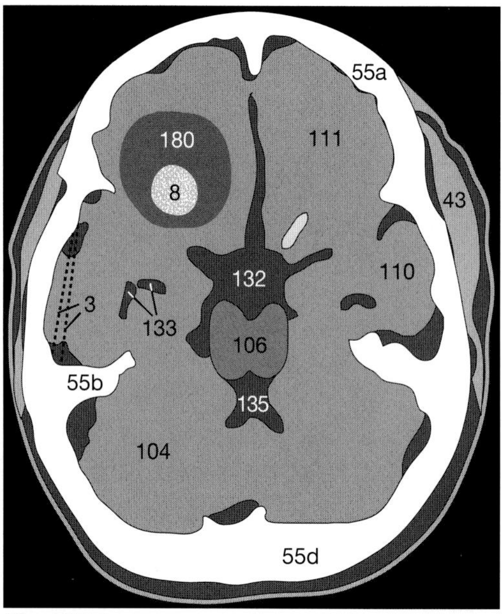

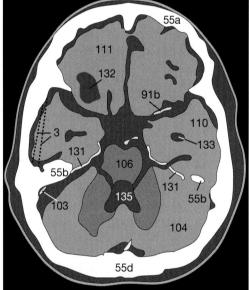

Fig. 52.1b

Bleeding Caused by a Contusion

As a direct consequence of skull trauma, cerebral contusion bleeding may occur (**Fig. 52.1a**). An acute hemorrhage (**8**) appears as a hyperdense mass which may be accompanied by surrounding edema (**180**) and displacement of adjacent brain tissue. In anemic patients the hematoma is less dense and may therefore appear isodense to normal brain.

If the vascular wall is damaged only secondarily by hypoperfusion mediated by edema, hemorrhage may not occur until hours or, more rarely, days after skull trauma. A CCT obtained immediately after skull trauma which does not show any pathologic changes, is therefore not a good predictor since delayed cerebral bleeding cannot be ruled out. A follow-up scan should be obtained if the patient's condition deteriorates. After complete resorption of a hematoma (**Fig. 52.2a**), a well-defined defect isodense with CSF remains (**132**).

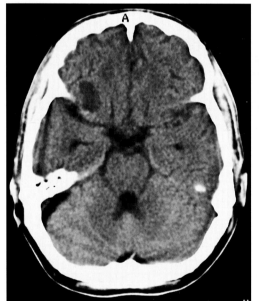

Fig. 52.2a

Fig. 52.2b

Contusion frequently leads to an epidural, subdural, or subarachnoid hemorrhage and may leak into the ventricles (**Fig. 53.1a**). Possible complications of such leakage or of a subarachnoid hemorrhage are disturbed CSF circulation caused by obstruction of the pacchionian granulations, the foramen of Monro, or of the 4th ventricle. An hydrocephalus with increased intracranial pressure and transtentorial herniation of the brain may result. Epidural and subdural hematomas can also lead to major displacement of brain tissue and to midline shifts. Quite frequently this in turn causes obstruction of the contralateral foramen of Monro resulting in unilateral dilation of the lateral ventricle on the side opposite the bleeding (**Fig. 54.3**). The characteristics useful in differential diagnosis of the various types of intracranial bleeding are listed in **Table 52.1**.

Type of bleeding	Characteristics
Subarachnoid bleeding	Hyperdense blood in the subarachnoid space or the basal cisterna instead of hypodense CSF
Subdural bleeding	Fresh hematoma: crescent-shaped, hyperdense bleeding close to the calvaria with ipsilateral edema; hematoma is concave toward hemisphere; may extend beyond cranial sutures
Epidural bleeding	Biconvex, smooth ellipsoidal in shape; close to calvaria; does not exceed cranial sutures; usually hyperdense, rarely sedimented

Table 52.1

If there is intraventricular extension of intracranial hemorrhage (**Fig. 53.1a**), physiologic calcification of the choroid plexus **(123)**, in the lateral **(133)** and 3rd ventricles **(134)**, as well as those of the habenulae and the pineal **(148)**, must be distinguished from fresh, hyperdense blood clots **(8)**. Please note the edema **(180)** surrounding the hemorrhage **(Fig. 53.1a)**.

If the patient has been lying supine, a horizontal fluid–fluid level caused by blood sedimenting in the posterior horns of the lateral ventricles may be seen (**Fig. 53.2a**). The patient is in danger of transtentorial herniation if the ambient cistern is effaced (**Fig. 53.2b**). In this case the 3rd ventricle is completely filled with clotted blood (➡ in **Fig. 53.2a, b**), and both lateral ventricles are markedly dilated. CSF has leaked into the paraventricular white mater (⇨). In addition, a lower section of this patient shows subarachnoid hemorrhage into the SAS (↙ , ↘ in **Fig. 53.2b**).

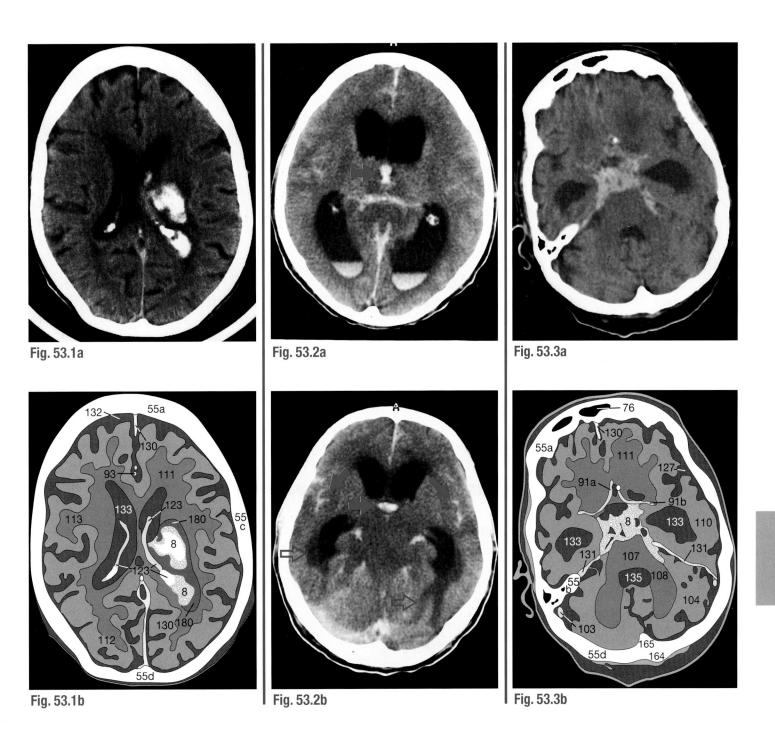

Fig. 53.1a   Fig. 53.2a   Fig. 53.3a

Fig. 53.1b   Fig. 53.2b   Fig. 53.3b

Subarachnoid Hemorrhage

An obstructive hydrocephalus, as caused by subarachnoid hemorrhage (**8** in **Fig. 53.3a, b**), may easily be identified because the temporal horns (**133**) of the lateral ventricles appear distended. In such cases it is important to have a closer look at the width of the SAS over the cerebral surface: blunted cerebral gyri usually indicate a diffuse cerebral edema. In the present case though, the width of the Sylvian fissure (**127**) and the surface SAS are normal. Acute edema is therefore not present (yet).

Since the surface SASs are very narrow in younger patients, it is possible to miss a subarachnoid hemorrhage in children. The only identifiable sign may be a small hyperdense area adjacent to the falx **(130)**. In adults a small subarachnoid hemorrhage also causes only a minor, circumscribed area of hyperdensity (**8** in **Fig. 54.1a**). At the time of this CT scan the bleeding was so slight that it had not yet caused any displacement of brain tissue.

Subdural Hematoma

Bleeding into the subdural space results from cerebral contusions, damaged vessels in the pia mater, or from torn emissary veins. The hematoma initially appears as a long, hyperdense margin close to the skull (**8** in **Fig. 54.2a**). In contrast to an epidural hematoma, it

is usually somewhat irregular in shape and slightly concave toward the adjacent hemisphere. This kind of bleeding is not confined by cranial sutures and may spread along the entire convexity of the hemisphere.

Subdural hematomas can also cause marked displacement of brain tissue (**Fig. 54.3a**) and lead to disturbances in CSF circulation and to incarceration of the brain stem in the tentorial notch. It is therefore not as important, for treatment purposes, to distinguish between a subhematoma or an epidural hematoma as it is to ascertain the extent of the hemorrhage. Hematomas with the propensity to expand, especially if edema is a threat, should therefore be drained or treated surgically.

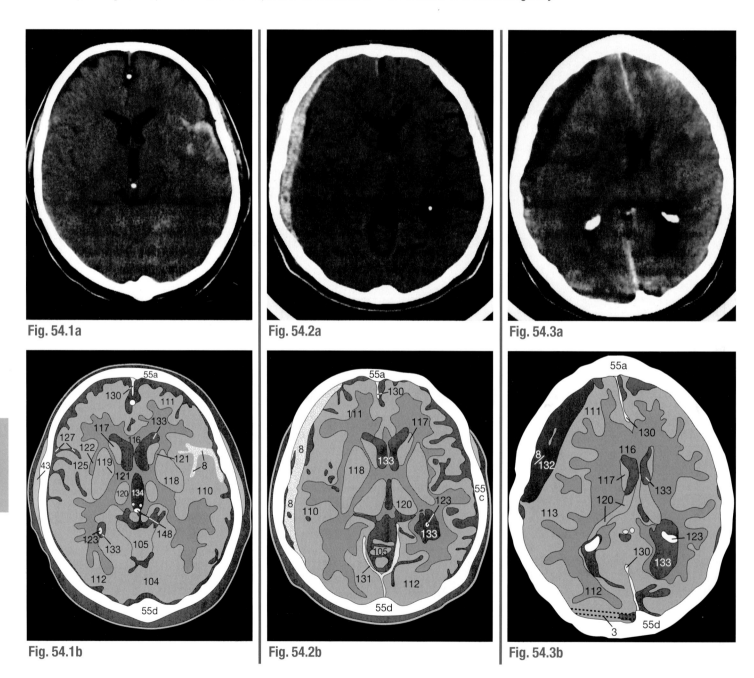

Fig. 54.1a

Fig. 54.2a

Fig. 54.3a

Fig. 54.1b

Fig. 54.2b

Fig. 54.3b

Chronic subdural hematomas (**8** in **Fig. 54.3a**) may appear homogeneously hypodense or show inhomogeneous density with sedimentation of blood. The danger involved in a small, venous bleed is the symptom-free interval and the slow onset of somnolence up to the development of a coma. Therefore, a patient with suspected bleeding after cranial trauma should always be kept under observation in order to detect any clinical deterioration.

Extradural Hematomas

Bleedings into the extradural spaces are usually caused by damage to the middle meningeal artery, and rarely by venous bleeding from the sinuses or the pacchionian bodies. Predisposed areas are temporoparietal regions or sometimes the posterior cranial fossa, in which case there is severe danger of tonsillar herniation. Arterial hemorrhage lifts the dura from the inner surface of the cranium (55) and then appears as a biconvex, hyperdense area with a smooth border to the adjacent hemisphere. The hematoma does not extend beyond the sutures between the frontal (55a), temporal (55b), parietal (55c), or occipital (55d) bones. In small extradural hematomas (8) the biconvex shape is not distinct (Fig. 55.1a), making it difficult to differentiate the finding from a subdural hematoma.

It is important to distinguish between a closed skull fracture, with an intact dura, and a compound skull fracture with the danger of secondary infection. An unequivocal sign of a compound skull fracture (Fig. 55.2a) is the evidence of intracranial air bubbles (4), which prove that there is a connection between intracranial spaces and the paranasal sinuses or the outside. It is difficult to determine whether the bilateral, hyperdense hematomas (8) in Figure 55.2 are extradural or subdural. In this case the distortion of the midline was caused by the right-sided, perilesional edema (left side of Fig. 55.2a) since it was shifted toward the left (the side of the hematoma).

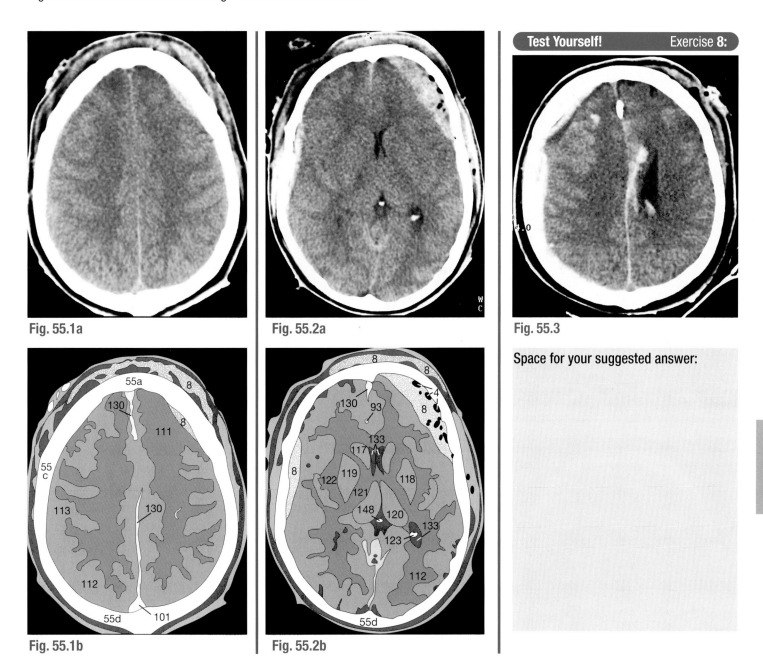

Fig. 55.1a

Fig. 55.2a

Fig. 55.3

Fig. 55.1b

Fig. 55.2b

Space for your suggested answer:

Test Yourself! Exercise 8:

Test Yourself! Exercise 8:
When looking at the image of another patient (Fig. 55.3) you will note several pathologic changes. Use the free space below the picture to note how many different types of bleeding (if any) you can distinguish and what other pathology/complications you suspect. You will find the answers at the end of the book, but remember: be a good sport and don't cheat, think first!

Apart from cardiovascular and malignant diseases, cerebral infarctions are among the most frequent causes of death. A thrombus occludes a cerebral artery, which leads to irreversible necrosis in the area of blood supply. Vascular occlusion develops in association with atherosclerotic changes of cerebral arteries or, less frequently, as a result of arteritis. A further cause are blood clots from the left heart or thrombotic plaques from the carotid bifurcation which embolize into a cerebral vessel.

In case of embolization, diffusely situated, small, hypodense zones of infarction in both basal ganglia and hemispheres are typical. Old emboli result in small, well-defined areas **(180)** which eventually appear isodense to the CSF **(132)**. Such areas are called lacunal infarcts **(Fig. 56.1a)**. A diffuse pattern of defects calls for color flow Doppler imaging or carotid angiography and an echocardiogram to exclude atrial thrombus.

Please remember that in a suspected stroke it might take up to 30 hours to distinguish clearly the accompanying edema as a hypodense lesion from unaffected brain tissue. A CT scan should be repeated if the initial scan does not show any pathologic changes even though the patient is symptomatic and if symptoms do not resolve (resolution of symptoms points to a **t**ransient **i**schemic **a**ttack, TIA). In case of a TIA no abnormalities are visible in the CT scan.

In contrast to the TIA, the **p**rolonged **r**eversible **i**schemic **n**eurologic **d**eficit (**PRIND**) is often associated with hypodense zones of edema in the CT scan.

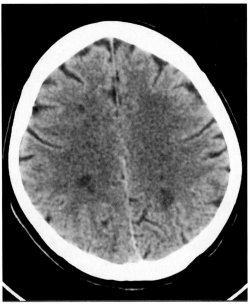
Fig. 56.1a

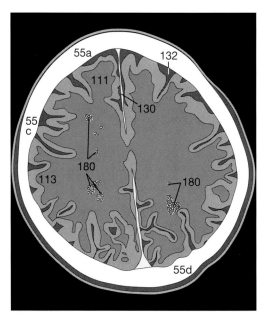
Fig. 56.1b

If the area of infarction corresponds to the distribution of a cerebral artery, then one should consider an occlusion of the corresponding blood vessel. In classical infarctions of branches of the middle cerebral artery, ischemia will cause a hypodense area of edema (◄, ✔ in **Fig. 56.2a**).

Depending on the size, the infarction may have severe mass effect and cause midline shift. Smaller areas of infarction do not usually show any significant midline shift. If the arterial walls are damaged, bleeding may occur and appear as hyperdense areas coating the neighboring gyri. The unenhanced follow-up CT scan in **Figure 56.2b** shows an additional bleed into the head of the right caudate nucleus (⇦) and right putamen (✖). In this case the infarction is 2 weeks old and necrotic tissue has been mostly resorbed and replaced by CSF.

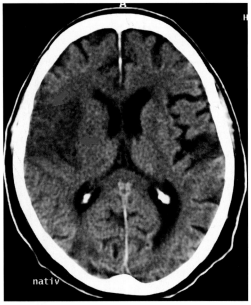
Fig. 56.2a

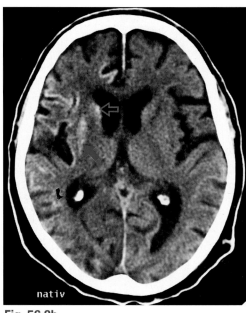
Fig. 56.2b

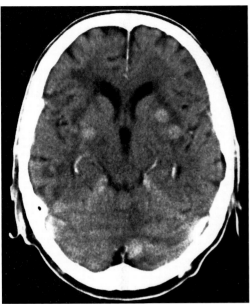

Fig. 57.1a

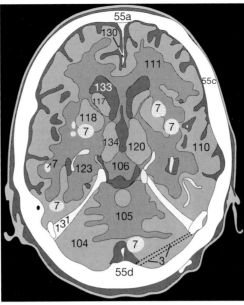

Fig. 57.1b

Whereas differential diagnosis (DD) of intracranial hemorrhage and infarction may be obtained without the use of CM, detection of cranial metastases **(7)** is definitely improved by the administration of i.v. CM. Even small areas in which the blood-brain barrier is disturbed become visible **(Fig. 57.1a)**. Large metastases sometimes cause surrounding edema **(180)**, which could be misinterpreted as infarct-related edema on unenhanced images if the metastasis appears isodense to the adjacent tissue. After i.v. CM the lesion in the left hemisphere **(7)** is clearly demarcated **(Fig. 57.2a)**. Did you also spot the second, smaller metastasis within the right frontal lobe, which also shows some surrounding edema **(180)**?

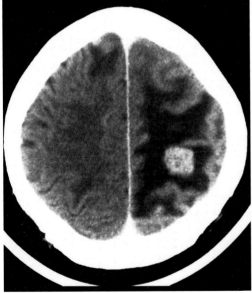

Fig. 57.2a

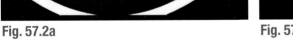

Fig. 57.2b

The differential diagnosis of brain tumors is made much easier by the injection of i.v. CM. In the unenhanced image **(Fig. 57.3a)**, the temporoparietal glioblastoma on the left **(7)** which has a central necrosis **(181)** could have been mistaken for cerebral infarction. The post-CM image, however, reveals the typical appearance of a glioblastoma with an irregular rim enhancement of its margin **(Fig. 57.3c)**.

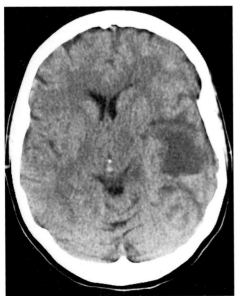

Fig. 57.3a

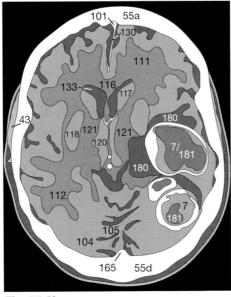

Fig. 57.3b

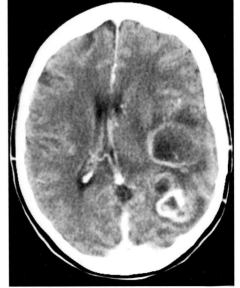

Abb. 57.3c

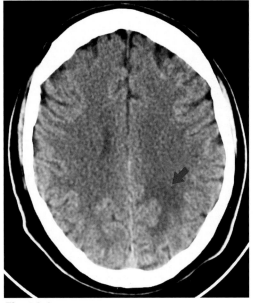

Fig. 58.1a

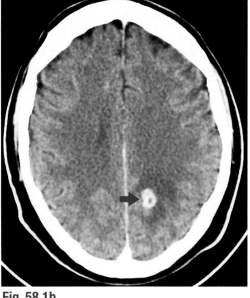

Fig. 58.1b

Another example of the advantages of i.v. CM is the demonstration of inflammatory processes, since the accompanying defect in the blood-brain barrier will not show on an unenhanced image. **Figure 58.1a** shows hypodense edema (✖) in an unenhanced section of a patient suffering from aortic valve endocarditis. Contrast medium **(Fig. 58.1b)** confirmed the finding by enhancing the inflammatory process (➡). Bacteria from the aortic valve caused this septic embolism in the left occipital lobe.

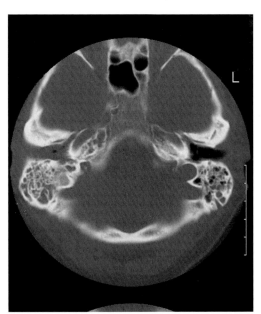

Fig. 58.2a

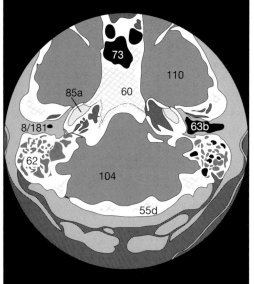

Fig. 58.2b

Inflammation of the paranasal sinuses and of the middle ear can already be diagnosed in native images as effusions **(8)**, for example in the normally air-filled mastoid cells **(62)**. Swelling of the mucous membranes of the external auditory canal **(63b)** is visible without the need for CM. **Figure 58.2a** shows bilateral otitis externa and media which is more severe on the right side where it involves the antrum and the mastoid cells. With progressing abscess formation an image on bone windows should be obtained in order to detect possible bone erosion.

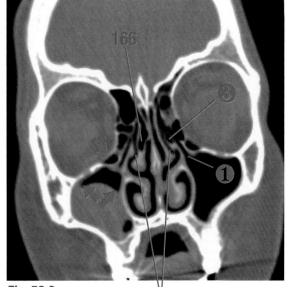

Fig. 58.3

A retention cyst, which often appears in one of the paranasal sinuses, should be considered in the differential diagnosis of advanced inflammations. They typically have a broad base on the wall of a paranasal sinus, extend into its lumen, and have a roundish convex shape (▼ , ➚ in **Fig. 58.3**).

Such cysts are only of significance if they obstruct the infundibulum (❶) of the maxillary sinus or the semilunar canal (❷), causing an accumulation of secretions. In patients with chronic sinusitis it is therefore important to check for an unobstructed lumen of the semilunar canal (❷) or for variations which may restrict mucociliary transport of secretory products.

Haller's cells (▼), a pneumatized middle concha **(166)** and a pneumatized uncinate process (❸) are among the most frequent variations. All of these variations can obstruct the semilunar canal and cause chronic, relapsing sinusitis.

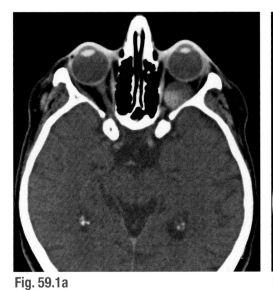

Fig. 59.1a

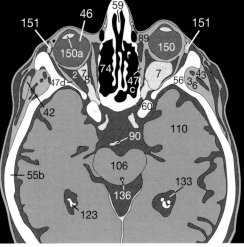

Fig. 59.1b

You have already seen pathologic changes in the lacrimal gland (pp. 37/38) and the CT morphology of an eye prosthesis (p. 49). Every mass within the orbit should, of course, be diagnosed early and treated effectively because of the possibly severe consequences to vision. In order not to miss tumor invasion into the walls of the orbit, bone windows should also be obtained. In **Figure 59.1a** there is a hemangioma **(7)** within the retrobulbar fat **(2)** which is not necessarily an indication for operation because of its benign character. In this case it causes a minor proptosis.

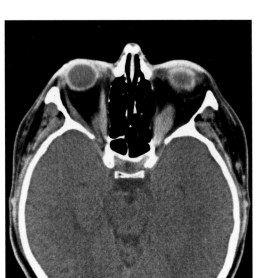

Fig. 59.2a

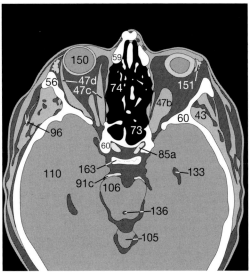

Fig. 59.2b

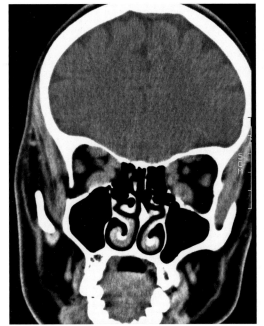

Fig. 59.3a

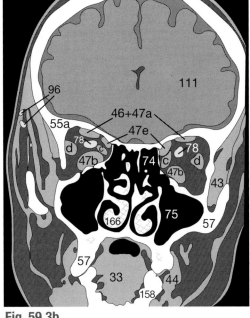

Fig. 59.3b

Endocrine Ophthalmopathy

Minimal discrete changes can be missed during the reporting of a CT scan: endocrine ophthalmopathy often appears as part of Graves' disease and can, in its early stage, only be diagnosed on the basis of a thickening of the external ocular muscles, e.g. the inferior rectus muscle **(47b** in **Figs. 59.2a, 59.3a)**.

Myositis should be considered in the differential diagnosis. If this early sign is not detected, the disease of the orbital tissue, which is most probably an autoimmune disease, may progress in the absence of therapeutic intervention. Therefore, you should always examine the symmetry of the external ocular muscles **(47)** when looking at an orbital CT scan.

There will often be a typical temporal pattern of involvement. The first finding is an increase in the volume of the inferior rectus muscle **(47b)**, the disease will continue and affect the medial rectus muscle **(47c)**, the superior rectus muscle **(47a)**, and finally all the other external ocular muscles.

In contrast to benign retention cysts (p. 58), malignant tumors of the paranasal sinuses often lead to destruction of the facial bones and may invade the orbit, the nasal cavity **(77)**, or even the cranial fossa. It is therefore useful to examine both the soft tissue and bone windows. For planning a resection, different CT planes might be necessary. The following example shows a tumor of the paranasal sinuses **(7)** in an axial **(Fig. 60.1a)** and a coronal view **(Fig. 60.2a)**. Originating from the mucous membranes of the right maxillary sinus **(75)**, the tumor has infiltrated the nasal cavity **(77)** and the ethmoid cells.

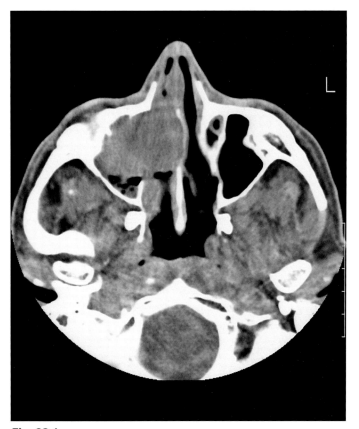

Fig. 60.1a

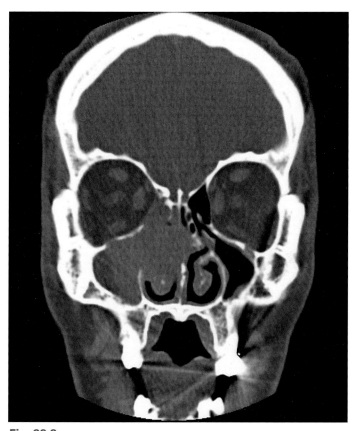

Fig. 60.2a

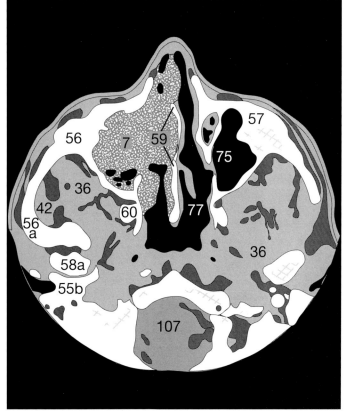

Fig. 60.1b

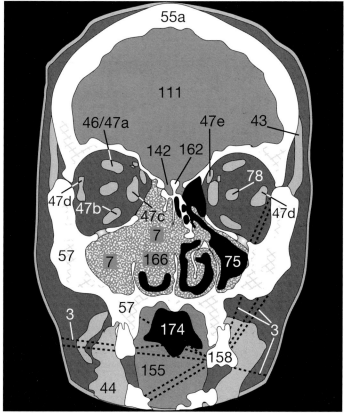

Fig. 60.2b

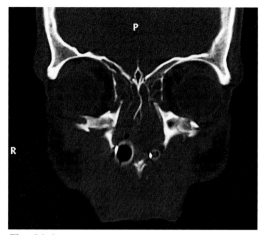

Fig. 61.1a

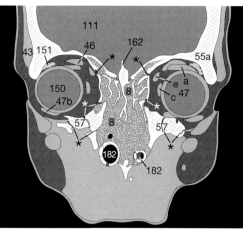

Fig. 61.1b

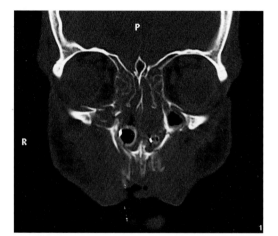

Fig. 61.2a

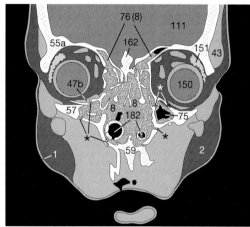

Fig. 61.2b

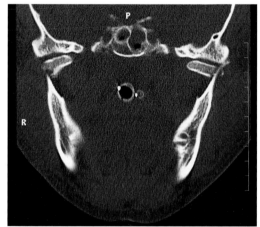

Fig. 61.3a

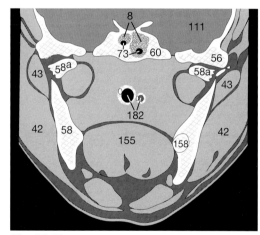

Fig. 61.3b

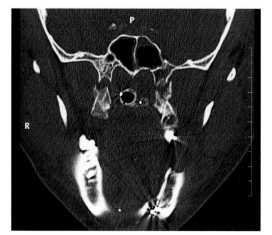

Fig. 61.4a

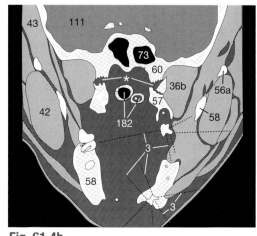

Fig. 61.4b

The most common reason for doing a coronal CT scan is, apart from determining the extent of chronic sinusitis, the diagnosis of fractures: in fractures of the orbital floor (**Figs. 61.1a**, **61.2a**) any accompanying herniation of retrobulbar fat (**2**) or the inferior rectus muscle (**47b**) into the fracture site (★) or even into the subjacent maxillary sinus (**75**) should be determined preoperatively. Diagnosis of the fracture in **Figure 61.2a** is easier because there are dislocated bone fragments. In addition, it is important to detect indirect signs of fracture, such as very fine, step-like contours of the bones and secondary bleeding (**8**) into the nasal cavity (**77**) or the frontal (**76**) and maxillary sinuses (**75**).

Another important question is whether or not the head of the mandible (**58a** in **Fig. 61.3a**) is fractured or the maxillary bone (**57**) has been fractured and displaced (★) from the sphenoid (**60**) bone (**Fig. 61.4a**). In this case severe bleeding (**8**) required intubation (**182**) and a nasogastric tube (**182**).

Fractures of the facial skull (Le Fort [33])

Type I Straight across the maxillary bones and the maxillary sinuses (Guérin's fracture)

Type II Across the zygomatic process of the maxilla, into the orbit, and through the frontal process of the maxilla to the contralateral side; maxillary sinus not involved

Type III Involving the lateral wall of the orbit and the frontal process of the maxilla to the contralateral side; ethmoid cells and zygomatic arch usually involved, sometimes also affecting the base of the skull.

Whenever there is no contraindication, CT examinations of the neck are carried out after i.v. administration of CM. Malignant and inflammatory processes can be depicted more accurately with the aid of CM. Adequate enhancement of cervical vessels requires higher doses of CM than, for example, in CTs of the head. In spiral CT, the injection of CM must be precisely timed to the acquisition of data. There are specific recommendations and suggested schemes for CM injection at the end of the manual.

Selection of the Image Plane

In an analogous manner to head CT, a sagittal planning topogram (scanogram) at lower resolution is obtained first. The transverse (axial) levels and gantry angulation are determined from this topogram **(Fig. 62.1)**. Usually sections of the neck are obtained using a 4–5 mm thickness. The axial images are obtained and printed as viewed from caudally so the right lobe of the thyroid is imaged to the left of the trachea, the <u>left</u> lobe to the <u>right</u>.

Images should be obtained with a small-scan field-of-view to optimize detail in smaller structures in the neck. As the thoracic inlet is approached during the scanning, the scan field-of-view is increased to include possible abnormalities in the clavicular fossa and the axilla.

Artifacts caused by dental prostheses **(3)** usually obscure surrounding structures (✱) in only one or two levels **(Fig. 62.2a)**. It may be necessary to carry out a second acquisition at another angle **(Fig. 62.2b)** to reveal areas hidden by artifact (✱).

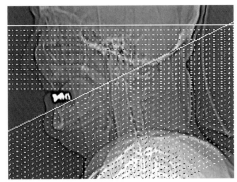

Fig. 62.1

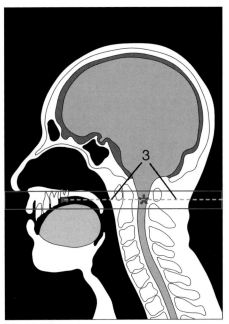

Fig. 62.2a

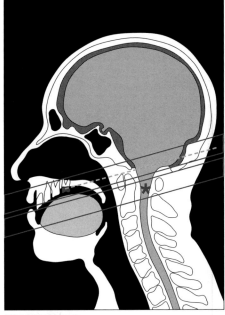

Fig. 62.2b

Systematic Sequence for Readings

We have already recommended a systematic approach with which to read CT scans of the head (see p. 24). For cervical CTs there is also no 'one and only' approach. The checklist presented here was developed through experience and is just one of many options for the beginner. Each examiner is free to set up his or her own checklist and strategy.

During neck imaging, separate hard copies at bone windows are rarely printed owing to cost. The radiologist must remember to check images at bone windows on the screen for fractures or lytic lesions.

Checklist for Reading Cervical CT Images

→ Symmetry of neck musculature?
→ Condition and clarity of fat?
→ Normal perfusion of vessels?
→ Thromboses or atherosclerotic stenoses?
→ Symmetry and definition of salivary glands?
→ Thyroid parenchyma homogeneous and without nodules?
→ Any focal pathologic enhancement with CM?
→ Narrowing of the tracheal lumen?
→ Assessment of lymph nodes? Number and size?
→ Cervical vertebrae examined in bone window?
→ Vertebral canal patent or narrowed?

The radiologist quickly reaches the limits of CT resolution (perhaps also of his/her anatomic knowledge) when trying to identify all of the different neck muscles. We have therefore reduced the amount of detail in the accompanying drawings so that smaller muscles are grouped. Single muscles have little clinical relevance and thus the legends to these images refer to combined muscle groups, e.g. the scalene muscles, the erector spinae muscles. Readers who want more anatomic detail should consult the relevant literature [5, 31].

Cervical images usually begin at the base of the skull and continue caudally to the thoracic inlet. The cranial sections **(Figs. 63.1–63.3)** therefore include the maxillary sinus **(75)**, the nasal cavity **(77)**, and the pharynx **(176)**. Dorsal to the pharynx lie the longus capitis and longus cervicis muscles **(26)** which extend caudally. Lateral to the mandible **(58)**, beginning in **Figure 63.2a**, the parotid gland **(153)** is situated next to the large cervical vessels and vagus nerve (also p. 64). In front of the pons/medulla oblongata **(107)** the vertebral arteries **(88)** join to form the basilar artery **(90)**.

The spread of inflammatory processes within the cervical connective tissue spaces is restricted within compartments defined by the cervical fascia [30]. The different layers of the cervical fascia are explained on the following page **(Fig. 64.4)**.

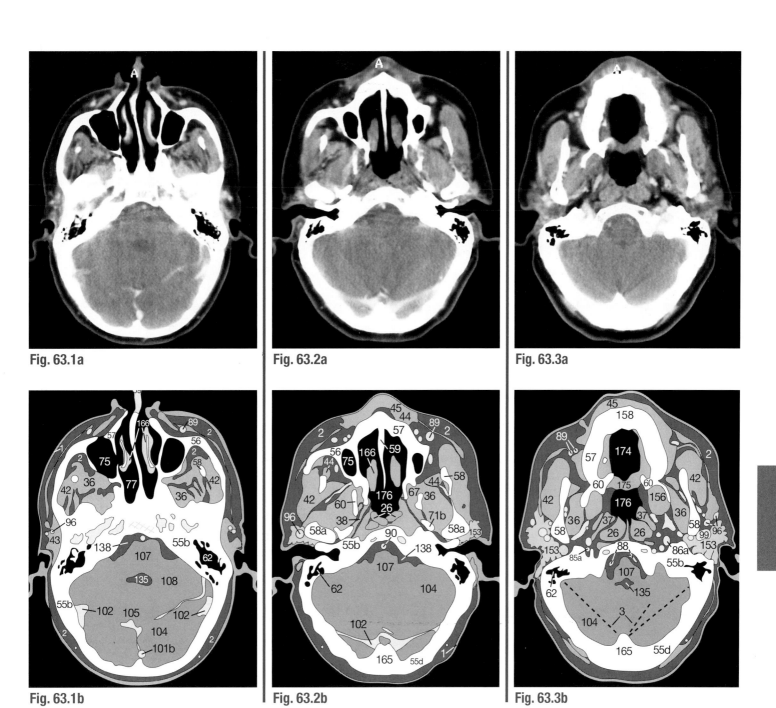

Fig. 63.1a

Fig. 63.2a

Fig. 63.3a

Fig. 63.1b

Fig. 63.2b

Fig. 63.3b

Further caudally the following cervical muscles become visible beneath the trapezius muscle (23): medial lie the semispinalis capitis (28) and longissimus capitis muscles (27), and more laterally the splenius capitis muscle (25). The parotid gland (153) is situated cranial and posterior to the submandibular gland (154) next to the mandible (58). The pharynx (176) is surrounded by Waldeyer's ring of tonsillar tissue (157, 156). Note that the carotid bulb is situated between **Figures 65.3a** and **65.4a**; it is the point at which the common carotid artery (85) bifurcates into internal (85a) and external (85b) carotid branches. Under the tongue (155) the floor of the mouth is organized in layers. From cranial to caudal are: the genioglossus muscle (33), further laterally the geniohyoid muscle (34), and the anterior belly of the digastric muscle (31). The thin superficial muscle is the platysma (48).

Compartments of the Neck

If infections or inflammatory processes originate in the suprasternal (⊕) or pretracheal spaces between the superficial fascia (✶) and the dorsal layer of the pretracheal fascia (✶✶), they cannot spread into the mediastinum because both fascias insert into the sternum (56 in **Fig. 64.4**). At the level of the parotid gland there is a similar barrier consisting of the sagittal septum which splits a retropharyngeal from a parapharyngeal space. Inflammations originating further dorsal, between the pretracheal (✶✶) and the prevertebral (✶✶✶) fascias, can spread caudally into the mediastinum.

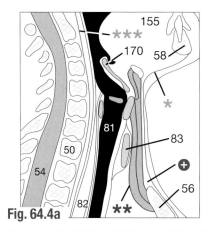

Fig. 64.4a

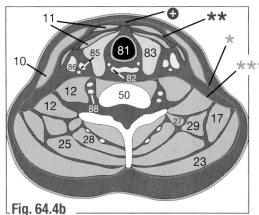

Fig. 64.4b

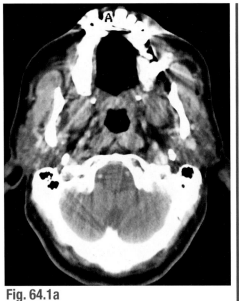

Fig. 64.1a

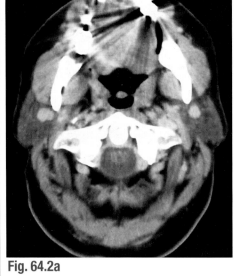

Fig. 64.2a

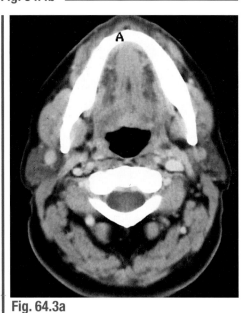

Fig. 64.3a

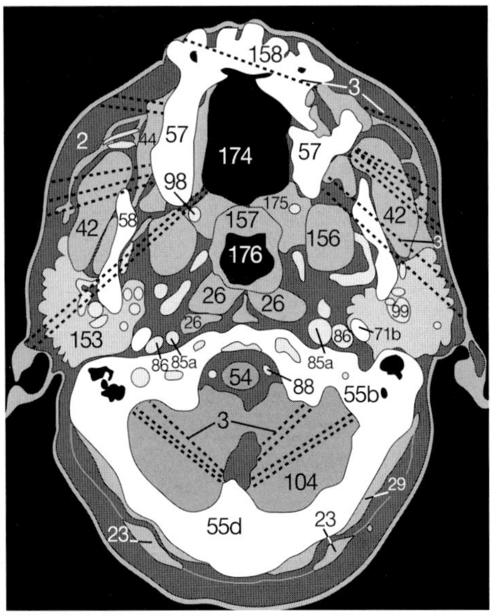

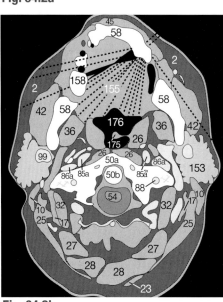

Fig. 64.1b

Fig. 64.2b

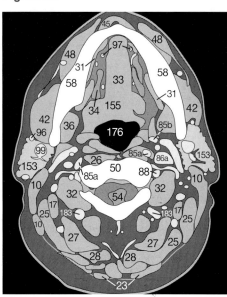

Fig. 64.3b

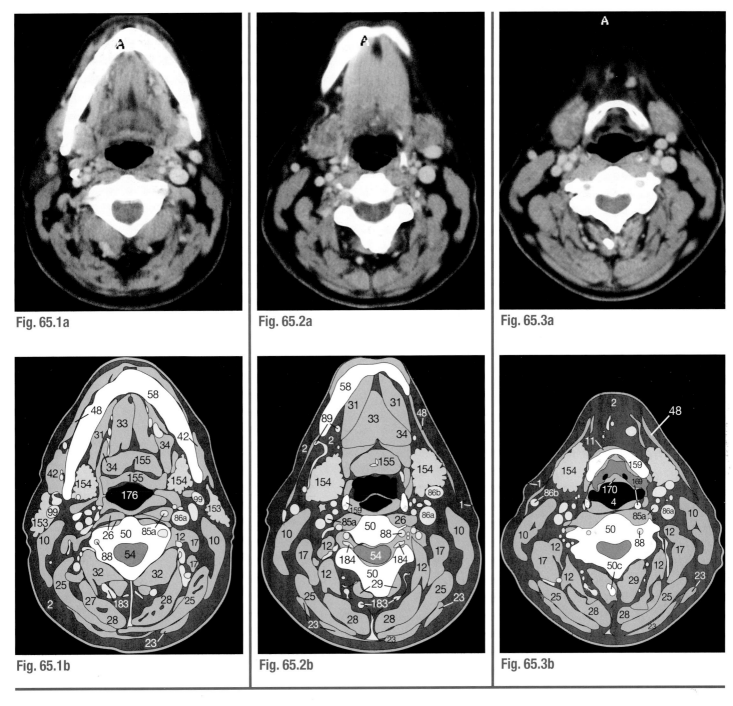

Fig. 65.1a

Fig. 65.2a

Fig. 65.3a

Fig. 65.1b

Fig. 65.2b

Fig. 65.3b

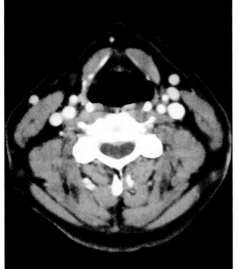

Fig. 65.4a

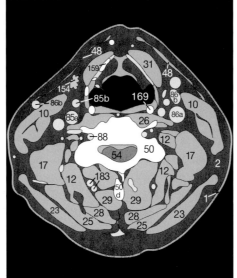

Fig. 65.4b

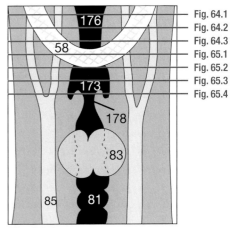

Fig. 65.5

The bifurcation of the common carotid artery (85) is an area of predilection for atherosclerotic plaques (Fig. 66.1a) which may be complicated by thrombus deposition (★). Note the positions of the cricoid (167) and arytenoid cartilages (168) at the rima glottidis (178). In these normal individuals CM enhances the density not only of the internal (86a), the external (86b), and the anterior jugular veins (86c), but also of the vertebral artery (88) in the transverse foramina of the cervical vertebrae. Always check for degenerative changes at the margins of the bodies of cervical vertebrae (50) or for herniated discs which might narrow the spinal canal containing the cervical cord (54). On either side of the trachea (81) lie the two lobes of the thyroid gland (83) which should have a smooth outline and have homogeneous parenchyma (Fig. 66.3a).

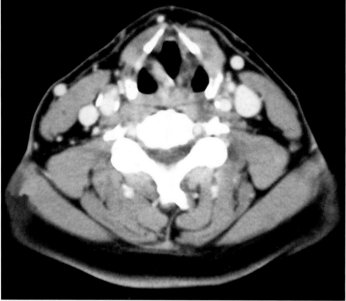

Fig. 66.1a

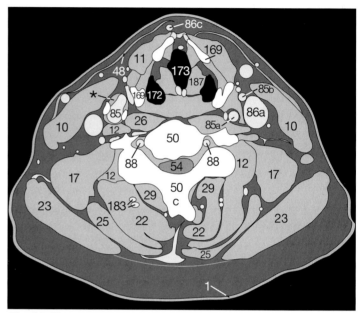

Fig. 66.1b

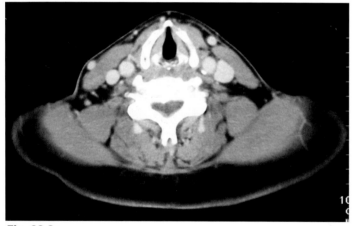

Fig. 66.2a

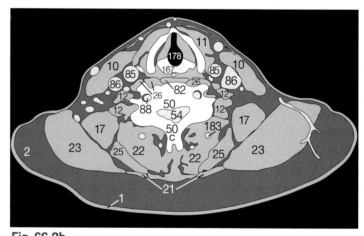

Fig. 66.2b

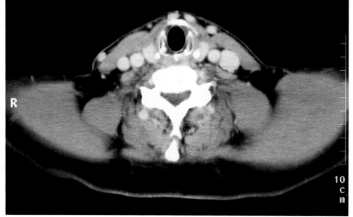

Fig. 66.3a

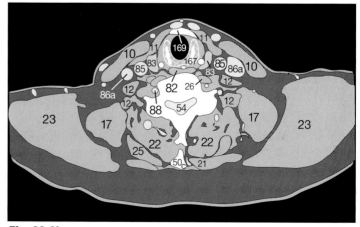

Fig. 66.3b

Because of its iodine content, the thyroid gland **(83)** appears hyperdense compared with surrounding muscles both before and, even more so, after the administration of CM (**Figs. 67.1–67.3**). Beginners occasionally mistake the esophagus **(82)**, dorsal to the trachea **(81)**, for swollen lymph nodes or a tumor. In case of doubt, comparison with other sections is helpful: usually a small, hypodense area indicates air in the lumen of the esophagus in an adjacent section. As a rule, the cervicothoracic junction is examined with the arms elevated to minimize artifacts due to bones. The muscles of the pectoral girdle as well as the shoulder joints therefore appear in unfamiliar positions. The following chapter deals with neck pathology and includes a short "Test Yourself"; images and drawings of normal anatomy extending further caudally are continued on page 72.

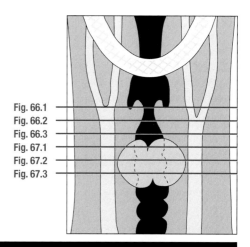

Fig. 66.1
Fig. 66.2
Fig. 66.3
Fig. 67.1
Fig. 67.2
Fig. 67.3

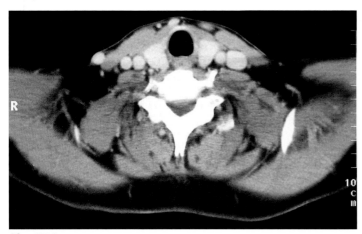

Fig. 67.1a

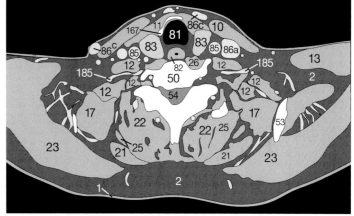

Fig. 67.1b

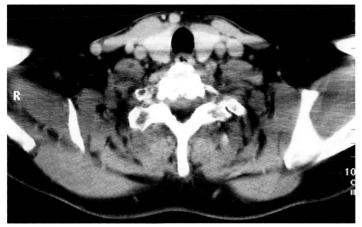

Fig. 67.2a

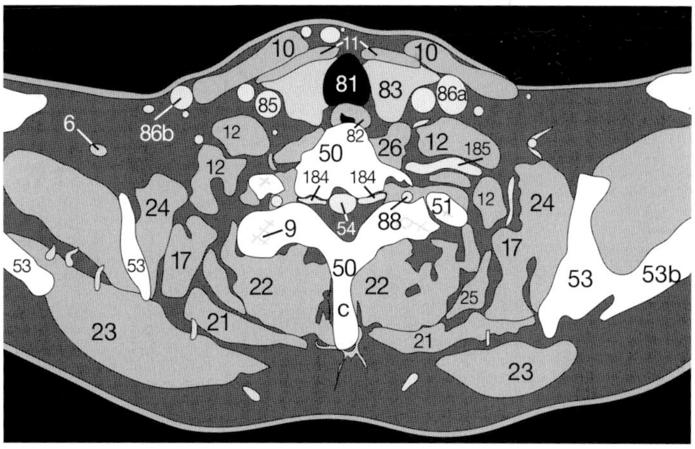

Fig. 67.2b

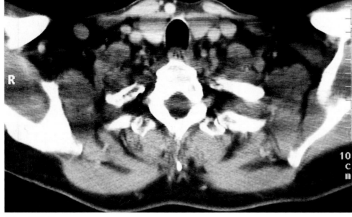

Fig. 67.3a

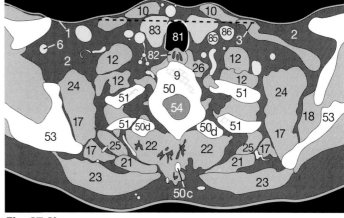

Fig. 67.3b

Enlarged cervical LNs (**Fig. 68.1a**) appear conspicuous as isolated nodular masses **(6)** that cannot be followed into adjacent levels (see p. 11). Large lymphomas **(7)** or conglomerate LN masses (**Fig. 68.1a**) often develop central necrosis **(181)**. It is sometimes difficult to distinguish them from abscesses with central necrosis **(181)** as shown, for example, in **Figure 68.2a**. Abscesses typically infiltrate the surrounding adipose tissue with a streaky pattern of edema **(180)** so that structures such as arteries, veins, or nerves (on the left side of the neck in **Fig. 68.2a**) become difficult to identify. In immune-suppressed patients, abscesses can become remarkably large. Compare the scans in **Figures 68.3a** (unenhanced) and **68.3b** (enhanced): after injection of CM, the outer wall of the abscess (**★**) as well as the central septa have become enhanced. These appearances are so similar to large hematomas or necrotic tumors that a differential diagnosis may be difficult without a detailed clinical history.

Note also the atherosclerotic plaques or thromboses in the lumen of the carotid artery **(85)** as in **Figure 68.1a**

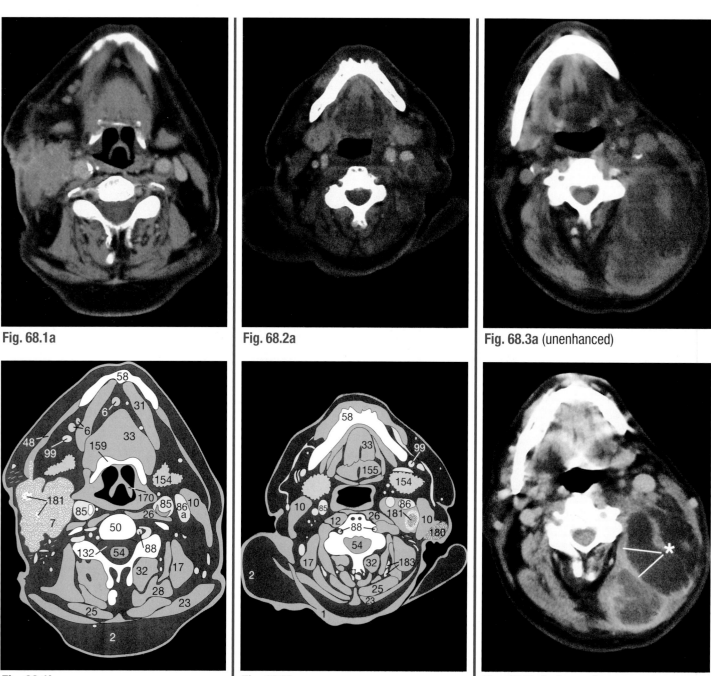

Fig. 68.1a

Fig. 68.2a

Fig. 68.3a (unenhanced)

Fig. 68.1b

Fig. 68.2b

Fig. 68.3b (enhanced)

The parenchyma of the thyroid gland **(83)** should appear sharply demarcated and have an homogeneous pattern in CT scans. The average transverse diameter of each lobe is 1–3 cm, 1–2 cm sagittally and 4–7 cm in craniocaudal direction. The total volume of the thyroid gland varies between 20 and 25 ml. If the thyroid is enlarged, check for tracheal compression or stenosis **(81)** and the caudal border of the goiter should be determined.

A benign struma **(83)** may extend into retrosternal regions and laterally displace supra-aortic vessels **(85, 87, 88)** **(Fig. 69.2)**.

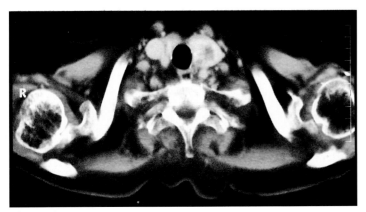

Fig. 69.1a

Fig. 69.1b

The parenchymal structure of a thyroid carcinoma **(7)** appears inhomogeneous, and the contours are not easily distinguished from the remaining normal parenchyma **(83)** **(Fig 69.1a)**.
In advanced stages of carcinoma **(Fig. 69.3)** cervical vessels and nerves are completely surrounded by tumor, and areas of necrosis **(181)** appear. The tracheal walls **(81)** are compressed and may become infiltrated. After partial resection of a struma **(Fig. 69.4)**, some thyroid tissue **(83)** may still be seen close to the trachea. In this case the left internal jugular vein was also removed and the lumen of the right one **(86a)** is therefore larger than normal.

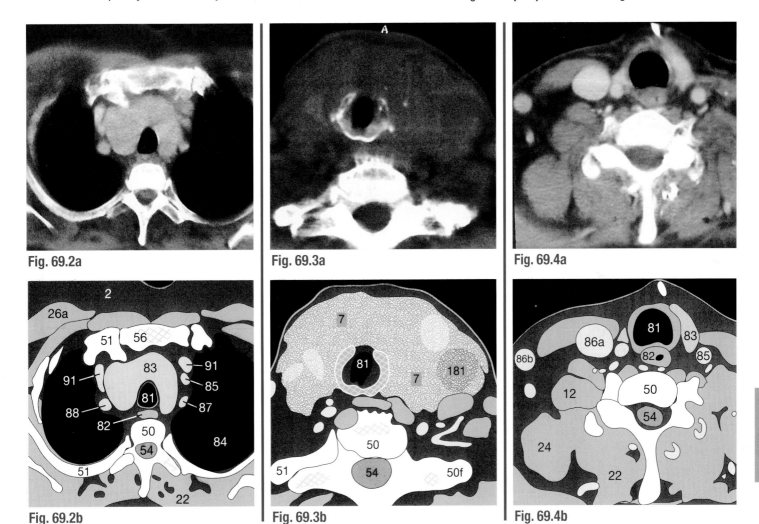

Fig. 69.2a

Fig. 69.3a

Fig. 69.4a

Fig. 69.2b

Fig. 69.3b

Fig. 69.4b

Before continuing to the next chapters, these exercises give you an opportunity to check your knowledge. The questions become increasingly difficult as you go along: the first question should pose no problems, whereas the last ones of each chapter will be a real challenge. Make the most of this opportunity for self control and take it in good grace if you find you missed something. In our experience these little tests will help you to remember better what you have learned.

It is much more effective to look up each gap in your knowledge as it occurs than to skip a problem and turn directly to the answer. You should therefore only turn to the answers at the back of the book when you have solved each problem by yourself. That way you will not see answers to questions you haven't tackled yet. It will keep you in suspense!

Exercise 9: Which window setting (window center and window width in HU) would you select for an optimal brain CT? Why? Before beginning the examination, what gantry angle do you choose for your slices in the planning topogram and what section thickness and section increments do you use? Why did you choose these settings?

Exercise 10: What do you remember about the criteria with which to distinguish the four types of intracranial hemorrhage? With which kinds of hemorrhage are you familiar? How can you differentiate between them in CT morphology? What complications or consequences must you particularly watch out for? (consult pp. 52–55 for help)

Type of hemorrhage:
-
-
-
-

Characteristics:

Exercise 11: How can you recognize a subarachnoid hemorrhage in children?

Exercise 12: Imagine the anatomy of the cerebral basal ganglia and then draw a transverse section at the level of the internal capsule. Compare your sketch with **Figures 28.2a** and **28.2b**. Repeat this exercise occasionally until you can do it with ease.

Exercise 13: Examine **Figure 70.1** carefully. The patient was involved in a car accident. Do not settle for the most obvious feature, look for other variations or abnormalities. What do you suspect?

Exercise 14: **Figure 70.2** contains an unusual variation; can you find it? After having noted it, look again to see whether you have really discovered all pathologic features.

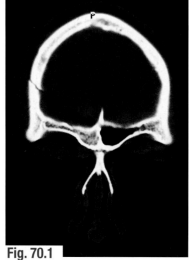

Fig. 70.1

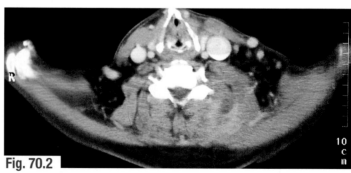

Fig. 70.2

Exercise 15:
The CCT in **Figure 71.1** is of a 43-year-old patient. Make a note of your tentative diagnosis and how you would proceed.

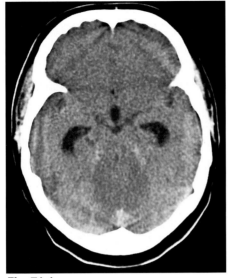

Fig. 71.1

Exercise 16:
Do you recognize anything unusual in **Figure 71.2**? Is there a pathologic abnormality? Or is it simply an artifact or even a normal finding?

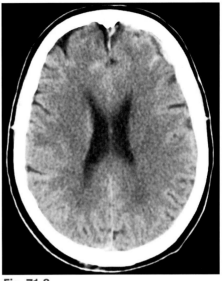

Fig. 71.2

Exercise 17:
Is there any feature in this orbital scan **(Fig. 71.3)** that would not be considered a normal finding? Note your observations below. Don't give up too quickly!

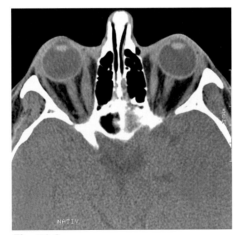

Fig. 71.3

Exercise 18:
A confused patient, from a home for the elderly, with suspected intracranial bleeding is brought in for a CCT. How many fresh hemorrhages **(Fig. 71.4)** do you see? What is your differential diagnosis? Which of them is the most probable diagnosis?
Which additional information could also be helpful?

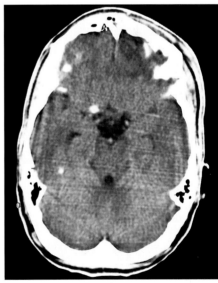

Fig. 71.4

Thoracic CT
72

After having discussed normal anatomy of caudal cervical sections (p. 67), normal thoracic anatomy is presented. From this page on you will find the number codes for the drawings in the rear foldout.

Selection of Image Plane

As a rule, the sections of the thorax are chosen in the transverse or axial plane at thicknesses and steps of 8 to 10 mm. Sections 10 mm thick will overlap by 1 mm, for example, when the patient table is advanced in 8-mm steps. A small topogram (Fig. 73.1) accompanying each sheet of images shows the position of the sections relative to the major anatomic structures of the region. In order not to miss any pathologic changes within the lung (review p. 13), it has become accepted practice to make a hard copy of both soft-tissue and lung windows. Each image can therefore be viewed at two different window settings. Again the large number of images necessitates a systematic technique for evaluation so as not to waste time looking randomly back and forth between them.

Systematic Sequence for Readings

The beginner often forgets to check the soft tissues of the thoracic wall because the examination of the mediastinum and the lungs is automatically considered more important. These tissues should

therefore be evaluated first. Common sites of abnormality are the breasts and fat in the axilla (2). After this–also using soft-tissue windows–the mediastinum is checked for pathologic masses. The easiest approach is to orient yourself relative to the arch of the aorta (89b), which can be recognized even by the inexperienced (Fig. 75.3). From this point cranially the major branches are identified to exclude pathologic masses in the upper mediastinum next to the brachiocephalic trunk (88), the left common carotid artery (85), the subclavian artery (87), as well as the brachiocephalic veins (91), superior vena cava (92), trachea (81), or more dorsally, the esophagus (82). Caudally, the most common sites for enlarged LNs are: at the aortopulmonary window, directly below the bifurcation of the trachea (81a), in the perihilar tissue, posterior to the crura of the diaphragm (= retrocrural) next to the descending aorta (89c). The presence of a few LNs smaller than 1.5 cm in diameter in the aortopulmonary window may be considered normal [19, 41]. Anterior to the aortic arch (89b) LNs of normal size are rarely seen in the CT. The evaluation of the soft-tissue window is complete when the heart (any coronary sclerosis, dilations?) and the lung hila (vessels well defined and not lobulated or enlarged) have been checked. Only now should the radiologist turn to the lung or pleural window.

Since the pleural window is very wide, the marrow of the spinal column as well as the parenchyma of the lung can be examined. It is therefore possible to evaluate bone structure in addition to the pulmonary vasculature. When examining the lung vessels, look for a gradual reduction in their diameter as you proceed from the hilum to the periphery. Pulmonary oligemia is normal only along the margins of the lobes and in the periphery.

It is essential to differentiate between cross-sectioned vessels and solid masses by comparing adjacent levels (cf. p. 11). More or less spherical solid masses may indicate intrapulmonary metastases. The checklist will help you read thoracic CTs systematically.

The simultaneous presentation of two window settings in one hard copy (both the lung and the soft-tissue window) has not proved practical because pathologic abnormalities which have density levels between the two would be overlooked. Consult the lung chapter on pages 101 ff. for scans in the lung window.

Checklist for Thorax Readings

1. On the soft-tissue window:

- soft tissues, especially:
  - axillary LNs
  - breast (malignant lesions?)
- mediastinum in four regions:
  - from the aortic arch cranially (LNs?, thymoma/struma?)
  - hilar region (configuration and size of vessels, lobulated and enlarged?)
  - heart and coronary arteries (sclerosis?)
  - four typical sites of predilection for LNs:
    - anterior to aortic arch (normal: almost none or < 6 mm)
    - in the aortopulmonary window (normal: < 4 LNs < 15 mm)
    - subcarinal (normal: < 10 mm; DD: esophagus)
    - next to descending aorta (normal: < 10 mm; DD: azygos)

2. On the lung window:

- Parenchyma of the lung:
  - normal branching pattern and caliber of vessels? vascular oligemia only at interlobar fissures? bullae?
  - any suspicious lung foci? inflammatory infiltrates?
- Pleura
  - plaques, calcification, pleural fluid, pneumothorax?
- Bones (vertebrae, scapula, ribs):
  - normal structure of marrow?
  - degenerative osteophytes?
  - focal lytic or sclerotic processes?
  - stenoses of the spinal canal?

Artifacts **(3)** will be observed at the level of the thoracic inlet if CM is present in the subclavian vein **(87)** at the time of data acquisition (cf. **Fig. 21.3**). The parenchyma of the thyroid gland **(83)** should appear homogeneous and clearly defined from the surrounding fat **(2)**. Asymmetry in the diameter of the jugular vein **(86)** is seen quite often and has no pathologic significance. Orthogonally sectioned branches of the axillary **(93)** and lateral thoracic **(95)** vessels must be distinguished from axillary LNs. If the arms are elevated, the supraspinatus muscle **(19)** lies medial to the spine of the scapula **(53b)** and the infraspinatus muscle **(20)**. Usually the pectoralis major **(26a)** and minor **(26b)** muscles are separated by a thin layer of fat.

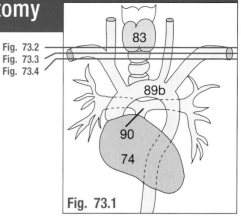

Fig. 73.1

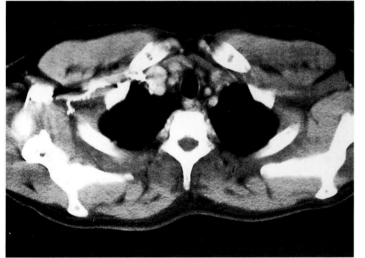

Fig. 73.2a

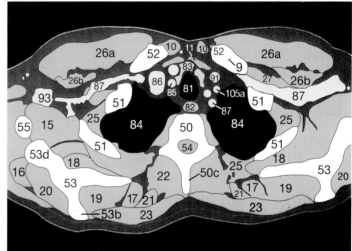

Fig. 73.2b

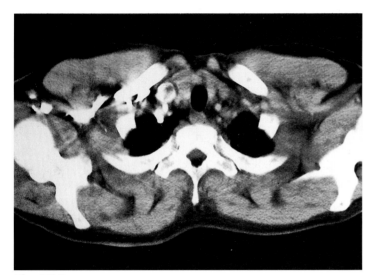

Fig. 73.3a

Fig. 73.3b

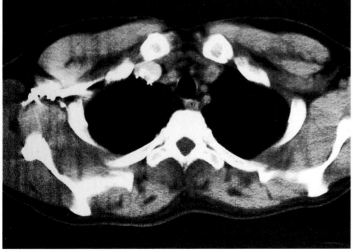

Fig. 73.4a

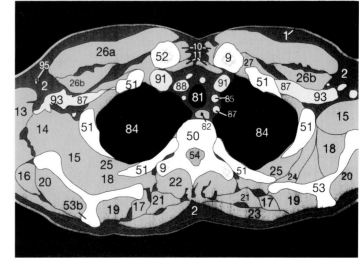

Fig. 73.4b

Thoracic CTs are also viewed from caudally. The left lung **(84)** appears on the right side of the image and vice versa. Beginning at the aortic arch **(89b** in **Fig. 75.2)**, the layout of the aortic arch vessels should be thoroughly familiar to you. At the section in **Figure 74.1**, the left subclavian artery **(87)** is seen most posteriorly and can be followed in cranial direction in the images on page 73. In front of the subclavian artery lies the left common carotid artery **(85)** and the brachiocephalic trunk **(88)**. More to the right and anteriorly are the brachiocephalic veins **(91)** which form the superior vena cava **(92)** at the levels of **Figures 74.3** to **75.1**. In the fat of the axilla **(2)**, normal LNs **(6)** are often recognizable by their typical indented shape: the hilum contains fat. At a different angle, the hypodense hilum will appear in the center of an oval. Healthy LNs are well defined and should not exceed 1 cm in diameter in this location (**Figs. 74.1** and **74.3**).

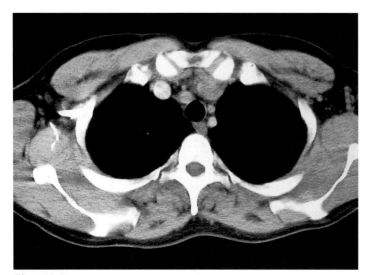

Fig. 74.1a

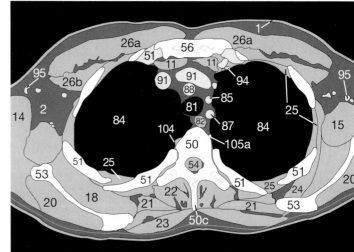

Fig. 74.1b

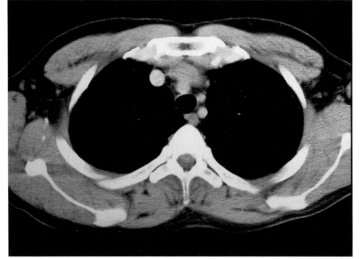

Fig. 74.2a

Fig. 74.2b

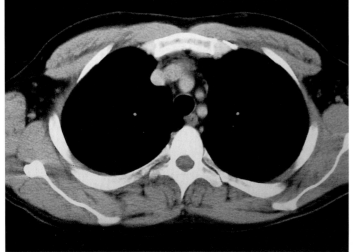

Fig. 74.3a

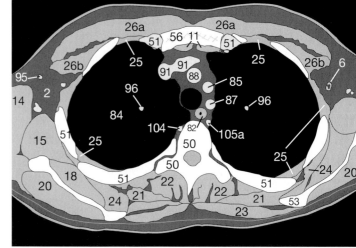

Fig. 74.3b

The azygos vein (104) lies dorsal to the trachea (81) next to the esophagus (82). Directly above the right main bronchus it arches anteriorly into the superior vena cava (92 in Fig. 75.2). Be sure not to confuse either the paravertebral azygos vein (104) nor the hemiazygos vein (105) and accessory hemiazygos (105a) with para-aortic LNs (Figs. 75.3 and 74.3).

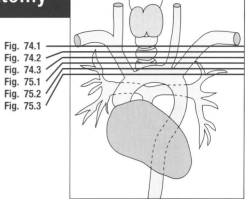

Fig. 74.1
Fig. 74.2
Fig. 74.3
Fig. 75.1
Fig. 75.2
Fig. 75.3

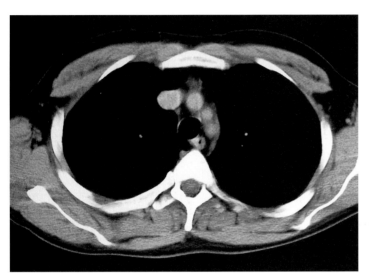

Fig. 75.1a

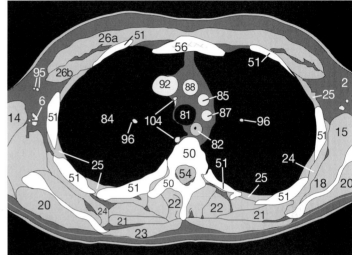

Fig. 75.1b

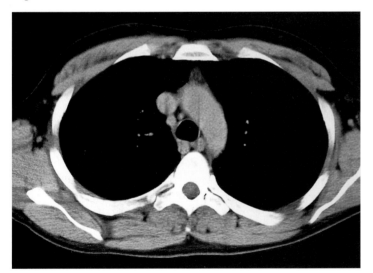

Fig. 75.2a

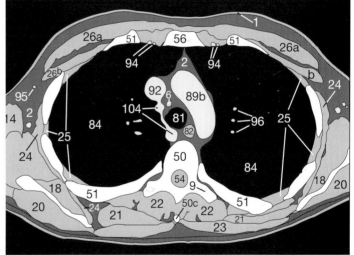

Fig. 75.2b

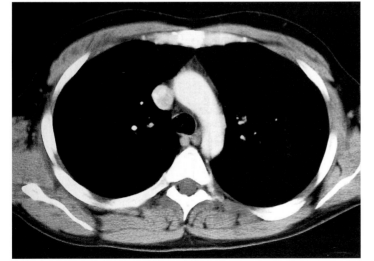

Fig. 75.3a

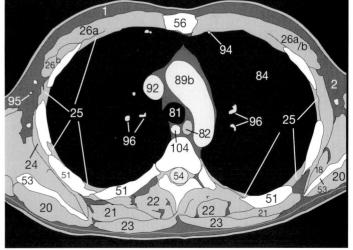

Fig. 75.3b

Immediately caudal to the arch of the aorta **(89b)** is situated the pulmonary trunk **(90)** which divides into the right **(90a)** and left **(90b)** pulmonary arteries. At the level of **Figures 76.1** and **76.2** there is the aortopulmonary window, a site of predilection for mediastinal LNs **(6)**. Also check for enlarged LNs or malignant masses in the subcarinal position between the two main bronchi **(81b)** close to the pulmonary vessels **(96) (Fig. 76.3)**. Near the internal thoracic (mammary) vessels **(94)** lies the regional lymphatic drainage of the medial parts of the breasts, whereas the lymphatic drainage of the lateral portions of the breasts is primarily to the axillary nodes.

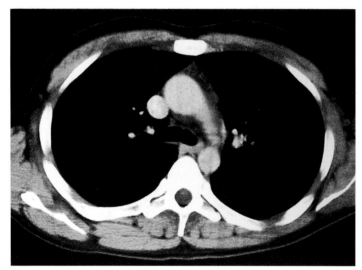

Fig. 76.1a

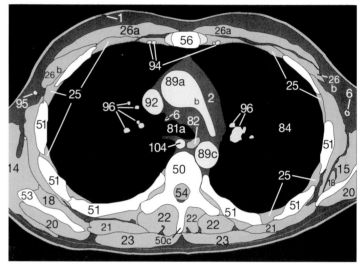

Fig. 76.1b

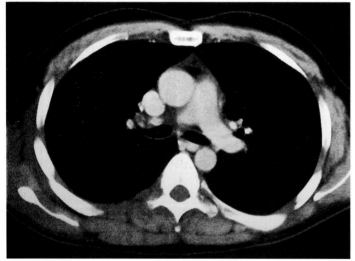

Fig. 76.2a

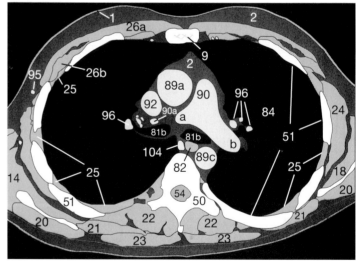

Fig. 76.2b

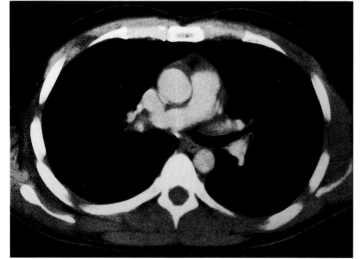

Fig. 76.3a

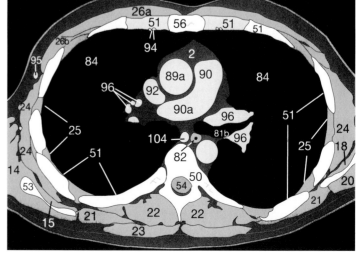

Fig. 76.3b

The glandular tissue **(73)** in the fat of the breasts of the anterior thoracic wall is easily differentiated from skin tumors because of the symmetry (**Figs. 77.1** and **77.2**). The main coronary arteries **(77)** are also distinguishable in the epicardial fat **(2)** (**Fig. 77.3**). Develop a clear mental picture of the positions of the azygos vein **(104)** and the esophagus **(82)** next to the descending aorta **(89c)** so that you will later be able to recognize any pathologic LNs close to these structures.

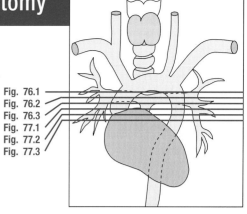

Fig. 76.1
Fig. 76.2
Fig. 76.3
Fig. 77.1
Fig. 77.2
Fig. 77.3

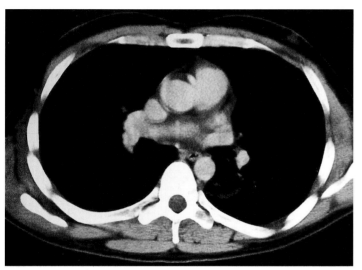

Fig. 77.1a

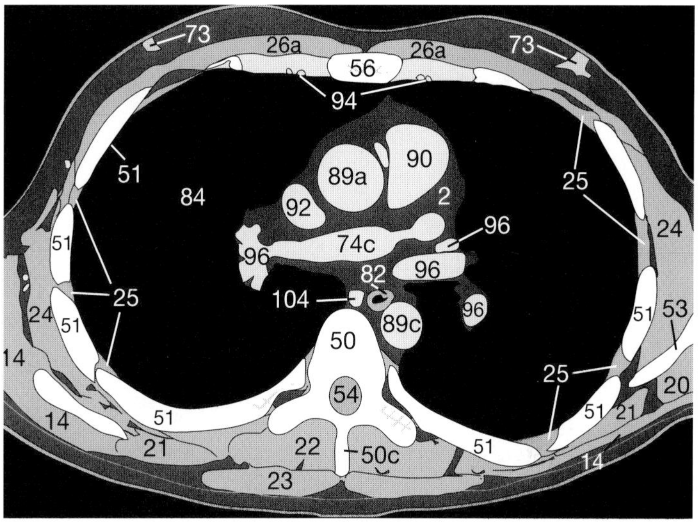

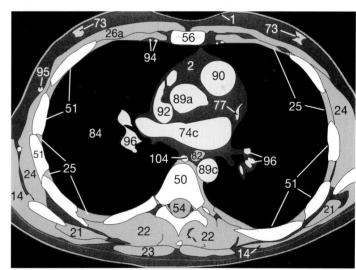

Fig. 77.1b

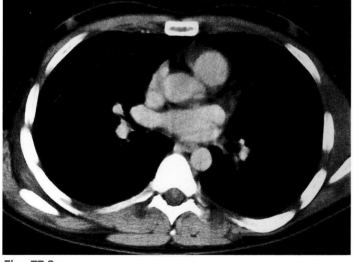

Fig. 77.2a

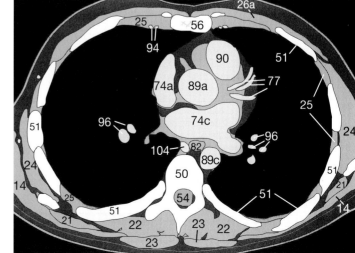

Fig. 77.2b

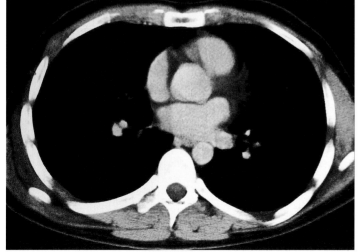

Fig. 77.3a

Fig. 77.3b

The left atrium **(74c)** is the most posterior chamber of the heart whereas the outlet of the left ventricle **(74d)** and the ascending aorta **(89a)** lie in the center of the heart. The right atrium **(74a)** lies on the right lateral side and the right ventricle **(74b)** anteriorly behind the sternum **(56)**. Only the larger central branches of the pulmonary vessels **(96)** can be seen on the soft-tissue window. The smaller, more peripheral, lung vessels are better judged on the lung window (not shown here).

Note the junction between the hemiazygos vein **(105)** and the azygos vein **(104)** which must not be confused with a paravertebral lymphoma **(Fig. 78.2)**.

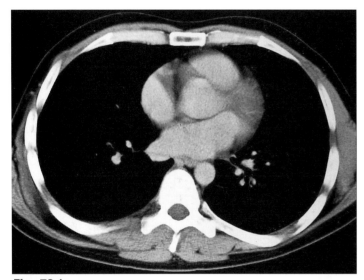

Fig. 78.1a

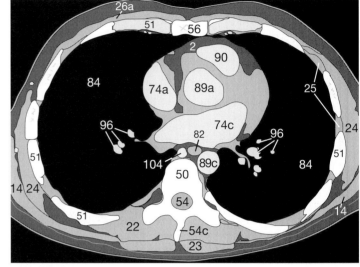

Fig. 78.1b

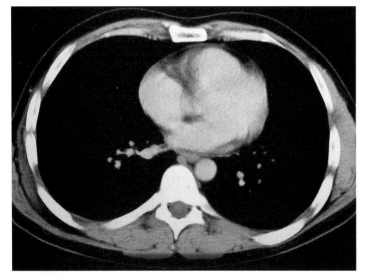

Fig. 78.2a

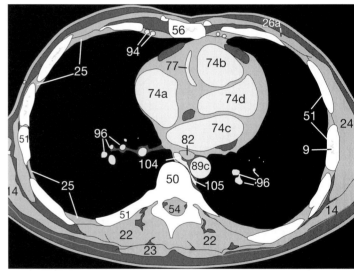

Fig. 78.2b

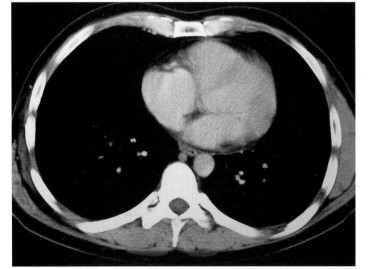

Fig. 78.3a

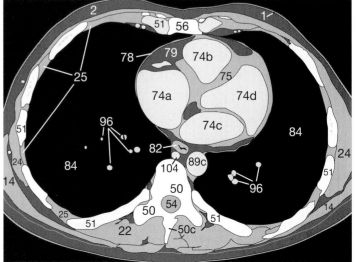

Fig. 78.3b

The sections on this page show the opening of the coronary sinus **(76)** into the right atrium **(74a)** and sequential sections of the coronary arteries **(77)**. The hypodense epicardial fat **(79)** must not be mistaken for fluid within the pericardial space. The internal thoracic artery, also known as the internal mammary artery **(94)**, is more and more frequently used in bypass operations. It is surgically anastomosed with the anterior descending branch of the left coronary artery.

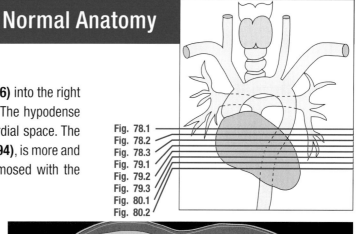

Fig. 78.1
Fig. 78.2
Fig. 78.3
Fig. 79.1
Fig. 79.2
Fig. 79.3
Fig. 80.1
Fig. 80.2

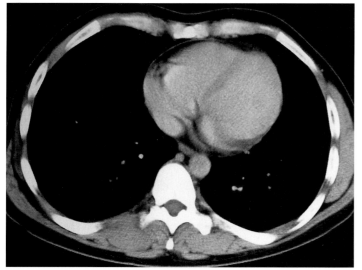

Fig. 79.1a

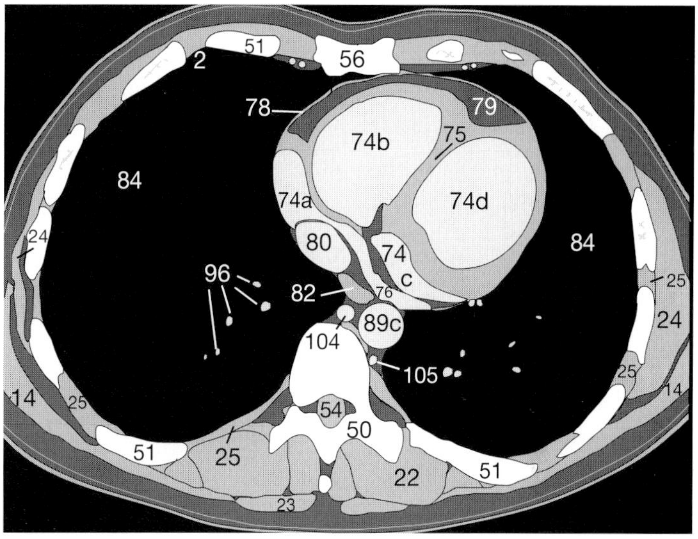

Fig. 79.1b

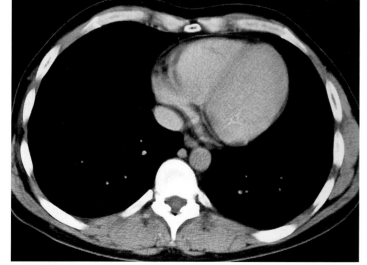

Fig. 79.2a

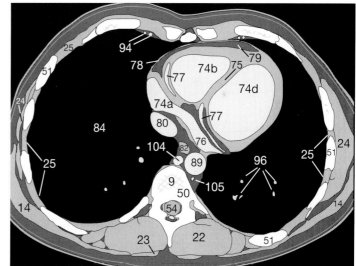

Fig. 79.2b

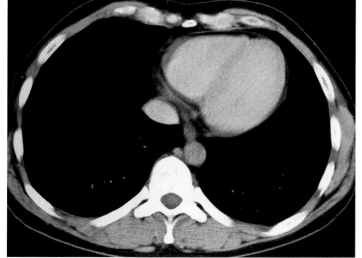

Fig. 79.3a

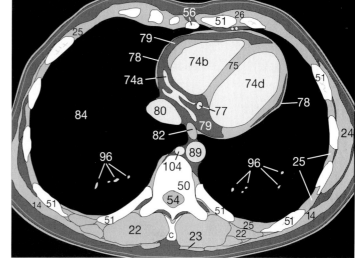

Fig. 79.3b

The inferior vena cava (80) is seen more caudally (Figs. 80.1 and 80.2), and finally the diaphragm (30) appears together with the upper parts of the liver (122). Many radiologists who suspect the presence of a bronchial carcinoma (BC) obtain images to the caudal edge of the liver (see p. 83) because a BC often metastasizes to the liver and the adrenal glands. The caliber of lung vessels near the periphery of the diaphragm is so small that they are not visible on the soft-tissue window, as in the present images. The pattern of the pulmonary vasculature should therefore be examined on the lung windows which include the negative density values of the Hounsfield scale. Only after this step has been carried out is the evaluation of a chest CT complete.

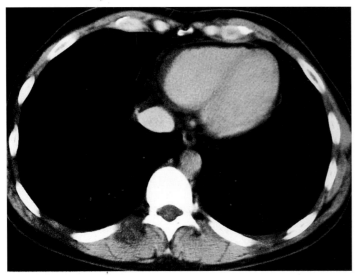

Fig. 80.1a

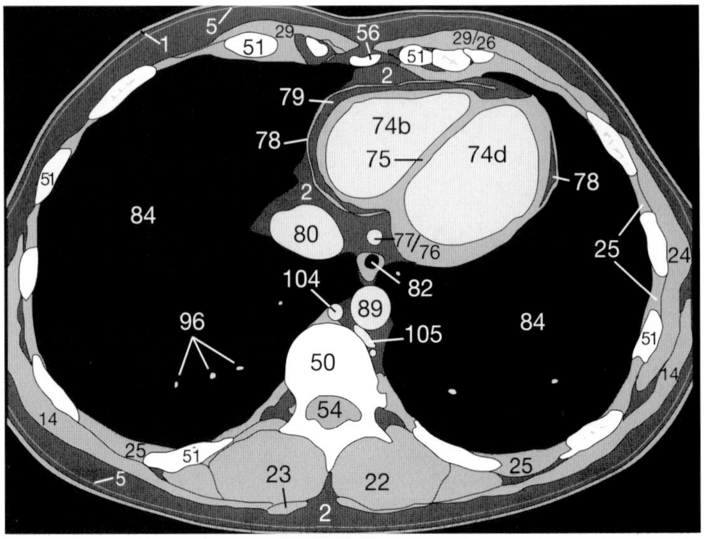

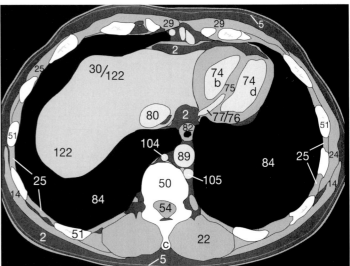

Fig. 80.1b

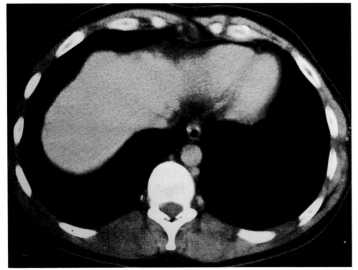

Fig. 80.2a

Fig. 80.2b

Test Yourself! Exercise **19:**

Write down a concise but complete sequence of all criteria for interpreting a thoracic CT. Then compare your notes with the checklist on page 72 and repeat this exercise from time to time until you remember every criterion.

In general, all soft-tissue organs should appear uniform and be well defined, except when partial volume effects occur (cf. p.10) or during the early arterial phase of CM enhancement in a helical scan (cf. p.122). Structures such as blood vessels and bowel loops should be clearly defined in intra-abdominal fat. The same applies to the fat in muscles. Poorly defined connective-tissue spaces may indicate edema or an inflammatory or malignant infiltration. If the anatomy cannot be clearly resolved, additional information can be gained by measuring the density of specific areas or by comparing unenhanced with CM-enhanced scans (cf. pp. 11 and 117).

Selection of Image Plane

The sections of the abdomen are also acquired transversally (=axially). If the table advance is set at 8 mm with a slice thickness of 10 mm, there will be an overlap of 1 mm on each side of the section. The small topograms on the following pages (based on **Fig. 81.1**) clearly show the slice positions as related to the anatomy of major structures for each series of images.

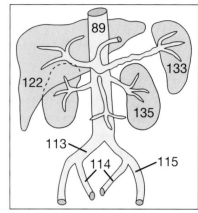

Fig. 81.1

Systematic Sequence for Readings

Analogous to interpreting chest CTs, we suggest you begin with the tissues of the abdominal wall. Considerable time is saved if you consistently look at them from cranial to caudal. For beginners a systematic inspection of each organ or system from cranial to caudal is recommended, so that you do not need to concentrate on too many structures at once. The proposed procedure encompasses two or three passages through the images. As you become experienced, you may wish to devise your own method. Experienced readers are more easily able to detect all pathologic changes in one passage from cranial to caudal.

It is sensible to evaluate internal organs that lie in the same transverse plane. The uniformity of the parenchyma, the size and the smooth surface of liver and spleen should be checked together. The same is true for the assessment of the pancreas and the adrenal glands: they also lie at the same level (cf. pp. 83/84). If the entire urinary system is to be examined, it saves time to inspect the reproductive organs and bladder in the lesser pelvis before looking at the cranial parts of the GIT, or the regional lymph nodes and the retroperitoneal vessels (see checklist on the right).

The presence of sclerotic and lytic bone lesions and the state of the spinal canal should be checked (cf. p.149).

Checklist for Abdominal Readings

Abdominal wall:	(especially periumbilical and inguinal regions) hernias, enlarged lymph nodes?
Liver and spleen:	homogeneous parenchyma without focal lesions? well-defined surfaces?
Gallbladder:	well-defined, thin wall? calculi?
Pancreas, adrenals:	well-defined, size normal?
Kidneys, ureter, and bladder	symmetric excretion of CM? obstruction, atrophy, bladder wall smooth and thin?
Reproductive organs:	uniform prostate of normal size? spermatic cord, uterus, and ovaries?
GIT:	well defined? normal thickness of walls? stenoses or dilations?
Retroperitoneum:	vessels: aneurysms? thromboses? enlarged lymph nodes? mesenteric (normally < 10 mm) retrocrural (normally < 7 mm) para-aortic (normally < 7 mm) parailiacal (normally < 12 mm) parainguinal (normally < 18 mm)
Bone window:	lumbar spine and pelvis: degenerative lesions? fractures? focal sclerotic or lytic lesions? spinal stenoses?

The images of the abdominal organs include the costodiaphragmatic recesses of the lungs **(84)** which extend quite far caudally, laterally, and dorsally. Liver **(122)** and spleen **(133)** parenchyma usually appear homogeneous without focal lesions in the venous phase of CM enhancement: branches of the portal vein **(102)** and the falciform ligament **(124)** can be distinguished. In order to assess the gastric wall **(129a)**, the stomach **(129)** can be filled with water which acts as a low density CM, after an i.v. injection of Buscopan. The diaphragm **(30)** between the thoracic and abdominal cavities has an attenuation similar to the parenchyma of the liver and spleen and can therefore not be differentiated from these organs if its thin dome is sectioned obliquely.

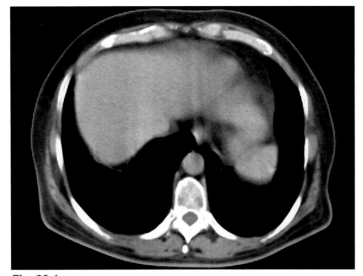

Fig. 82.1a

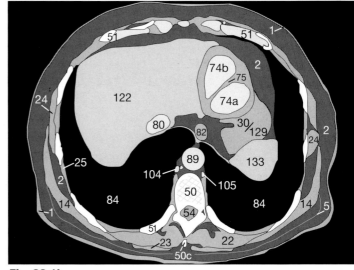

Fig. 82.1b

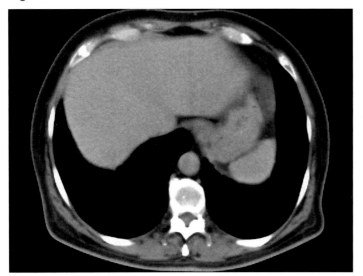

Fig. 82.2a

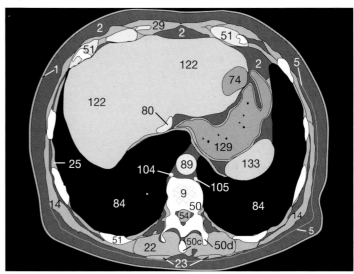

Fig. 82.2b

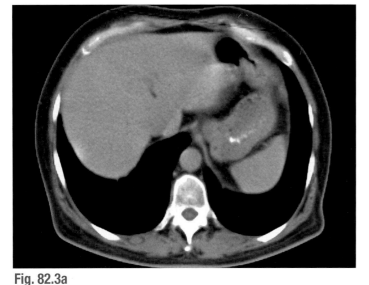

Fig. 82.3a

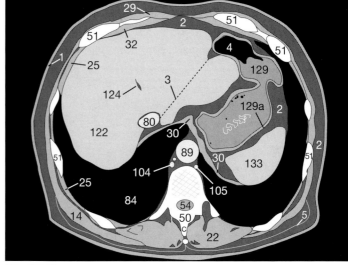

Fig. 82.3b

The right adrenal gland usually lies cranial to the upper pole of the kidney **(135)**, whereas the left adrenal gland lies ventral to the upper pole of the kidney. As a rule the two adrenal glands **(134)** are seen on the same sections. Note the position of the diaphragm **(30)** between the lung **(84)** and the inferior vena cava **(80)**. The vessels on the lesser curvature of the stomach **(109)** and the gastric walls **(129a)** are usually well defined and clearly demarcated in the surrounding fat and connective tissue **(2)**.

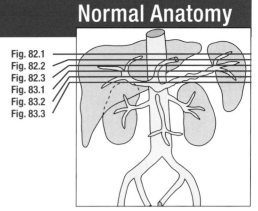

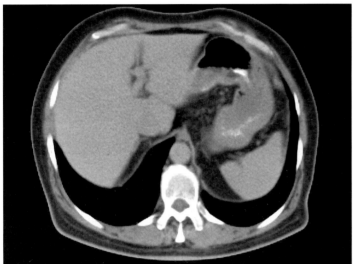

Fig. 83.1a

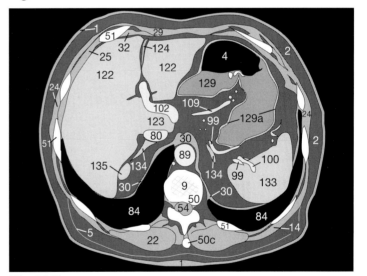

Fig. 83.1b

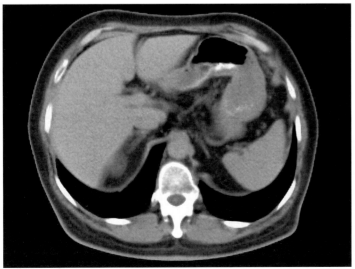

Fig. 83.2a

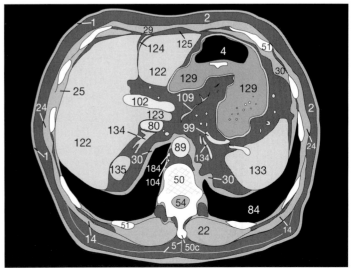

Fig. 83.2b

Fig. 83.3a

Fig. 83.3b

Typically the pancreas **(131)** has well-defined parenchyma with an irregular outline. The head and uncinate process of the pancreas extend quite far caudally (down to **Fig. 85.2**). The left adrenal gland **(134)** is often Y-shaped, whereas the right adrenal gland may look like an arrow or a comma. Note the origin of the celiac trunk **(97)** and the SMA **(106)** from the abdominal aorta **(89)**. Enlarged lymph nodes may frequently be found in this vicinity. In **Figure 84.3** the contrast-enhancing effect of an arterial bolus of CM becomes evident. At this point the SMA **(106)** has enhanced more than the accompanying vein **(107)** which does not contain any CM. Within moments **(Fig. 85.1)** the bolus of CM has also opacified the superior mesenteric vein **(107)**.

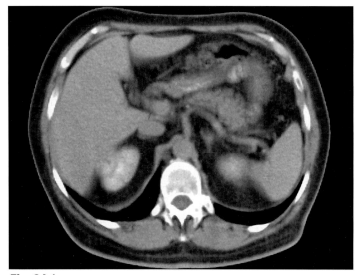

Fig. 84.1a

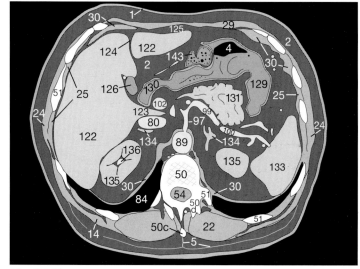

Fig. 84.1b

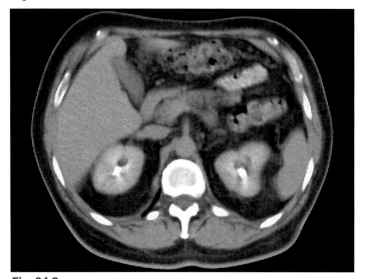

Fig. 84.2a

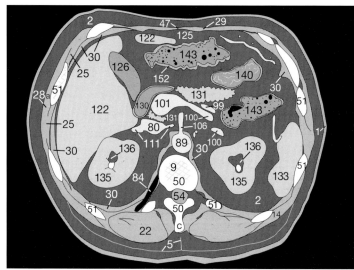

Fig. 84.2b

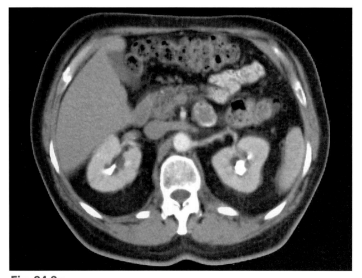

Fig. 84.3a

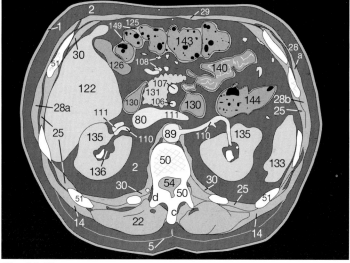

Fig. 84.3b

Look for arterial calcifications in the origins of the renal arteries **(110)** at the level of the renal veins **(111)**. The left renal vein does not always pass between the aorta **(89)** and the SMA **(106)** to the inferior vena cava **(80)**, as it does in **Figure 85.1**. Anatomic variations are not unusual (cf. p.112). Benign cysts **(169)** frequently occur in the renal pelvis **(136)** next to the ureter **(137)** or in the renal parenchyma **(135)** **(Figs. 85.2 and 85.3)**. Such cysts do <u>not</u> enhance after CM injection (cf. p.127).

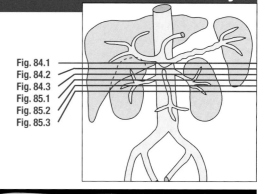

Fig. 84.1
Fig. 84.2
Fig. 84.3
Fig. 85.1
Fig. 85.2
Fig. 85.3

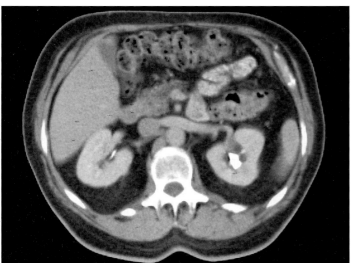

Fig. 85.1a

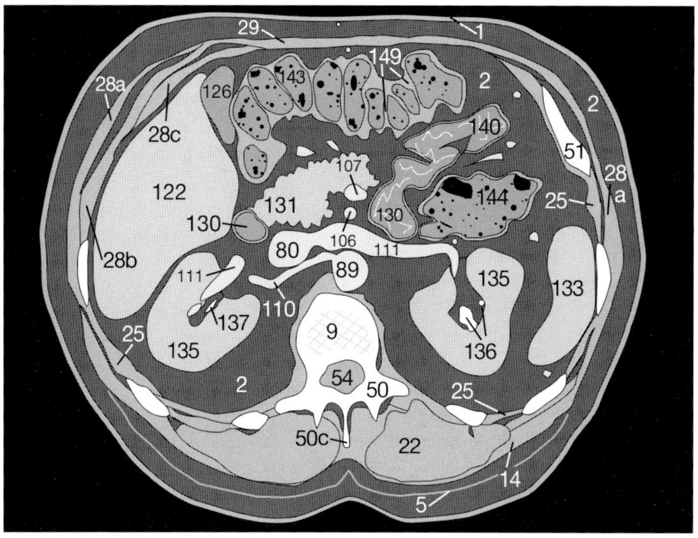

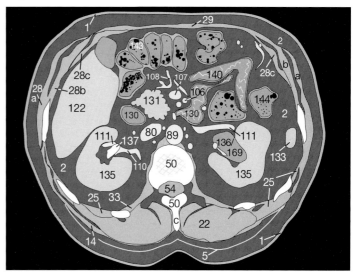

Fig. 85.1b

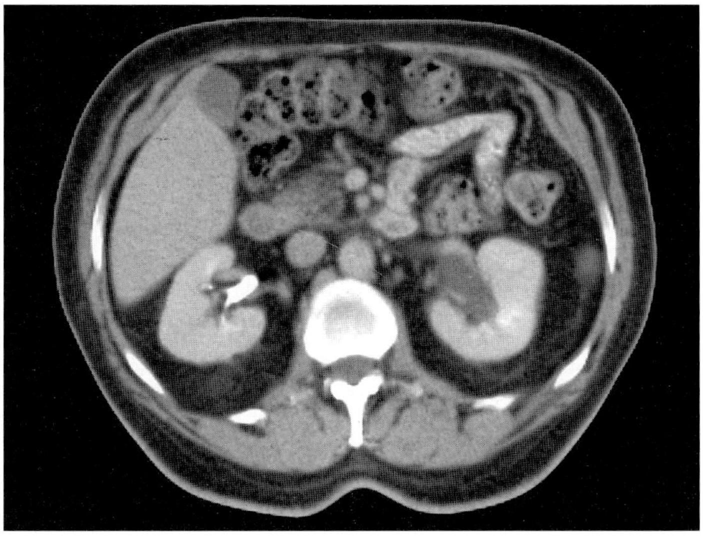

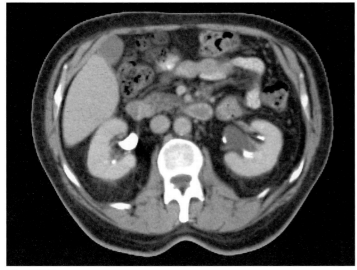

Fig. 85.2a

Fig. 85.2b

Fig. 85.3a

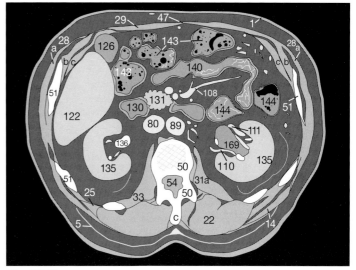

Fig. 85.3b

Close to the gallbladder **(126)** you can sometimes see partial volume effects **(Fig. 86.1)** of the adjacent colon **(143/144)**, the walls of which **(152)** should normally be thin and well defined in contrast to the root of the small bowel mesentery (as in **Fig. 86.3**). The duodenum **(130)** can only be distinguished from the other intestinal loops **(140)** on the basis of its position. At this level you should also check the kidneys **(135)** for smooth margins and possible parenchymal scarring. The presence of fat makes it easier to identify the rectus abdominis muscle **(29)** as well as the oblique muscles of the abdominal wall **(28a–c)**.

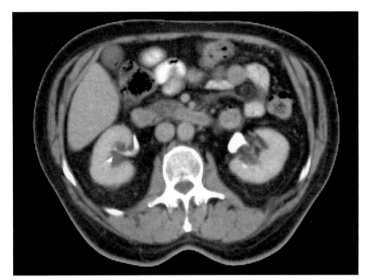

Fig. 86.1a

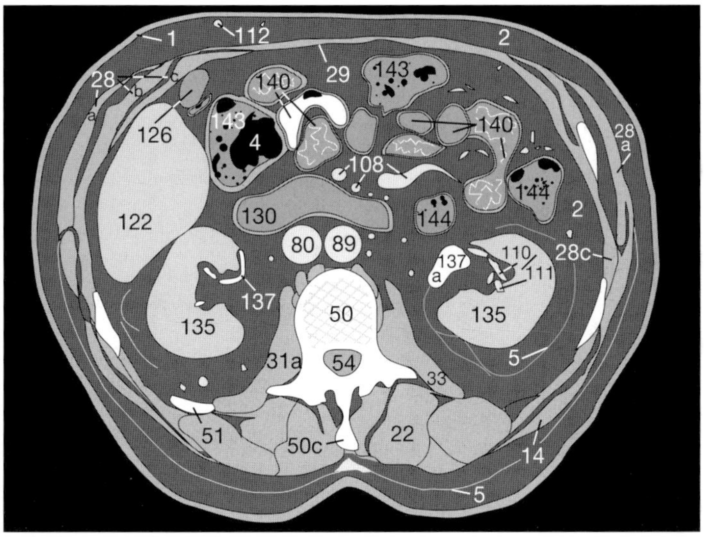

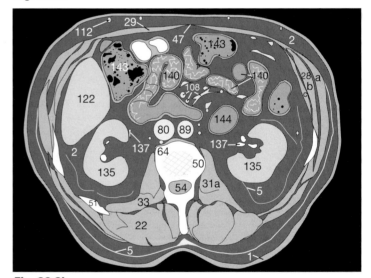

Fig. 86.1b

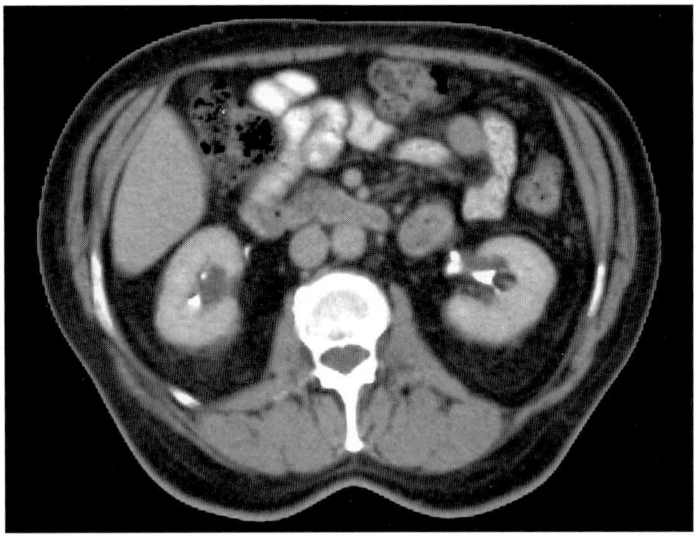

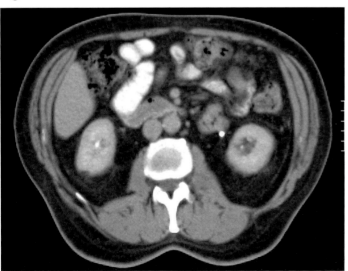

Fig. 86.2a

Fig. 86.2b

Fig. 86.3a

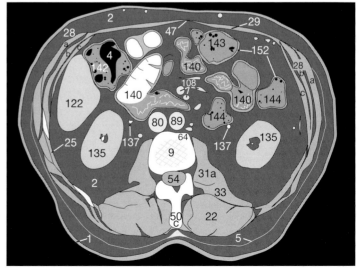

Fig. 86.3b

Note the typical position of the proximal parts of the ureters **(137)**, medial to the inferior poles of the kidneys **(135)** and anterior to the psoas muscle **(31a)**. In **Figures 87.2** and **87.3** the lumina of both ureters appear hyperdense because CM is being excreted in the urine. Parts of the renal fascia **(5)** can be identified in **Figures 87.2** and **87.3**. Haustrations caused by the semilunar folds (haustral folds) **(149)** are typical of the colon **(142–144** in the figures below).

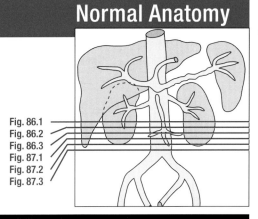

Fig. 86.1
Fig. 86.2
Fig. 86.3
Fig. 87.1
Fig. 87.2
Fig. 87.3

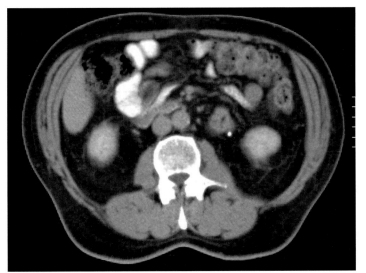

Fig. 87.1a

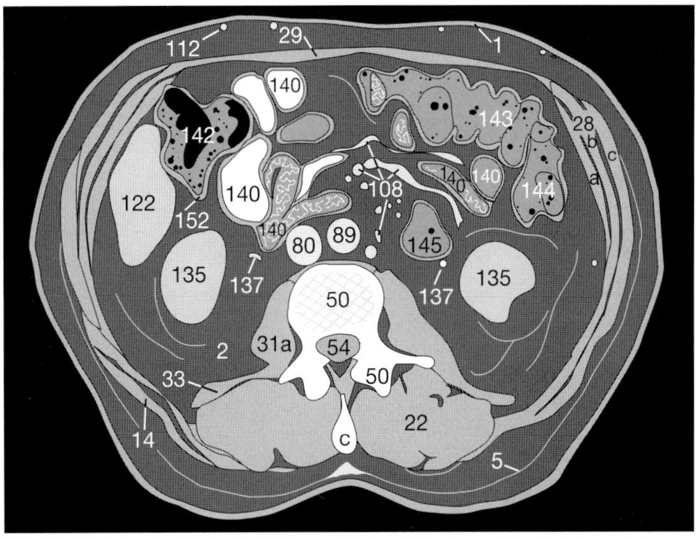

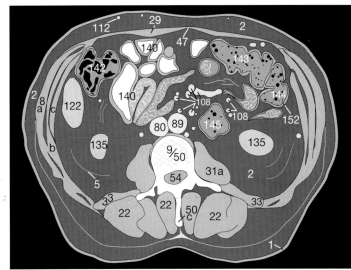

Fig. 87.1b

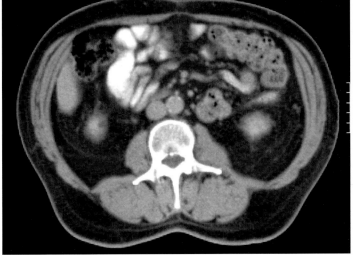

Fig. 87.2a

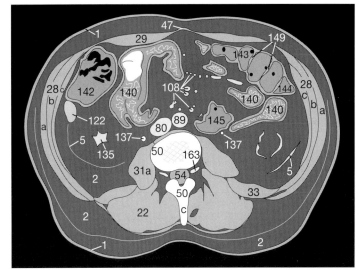

Fig. 87.2b

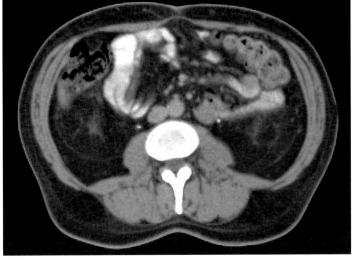

Fig. 87.3a

Fig. 87.3b

In **Figure 88.1**, the branching pattern of the superior mesenteric vessels **(108)** which supply the small bowel **(140)** can be seen. At the bifurcation of the aorta **(89)** (usually at L4 vertebral body, **Fig. 88.2**), the common iliac arteries **(113)** are anterior to the corresponding veins **(116)**. The two ureters **(137)** are located more laterally in front of the psoas muscles **(31a)**. Along with the iliac bones **(58)** the gluteus medius muscles **(35a)** appear and sometimes contain calcified intramuscular injections sites (cf. **Fig. 113.3**).

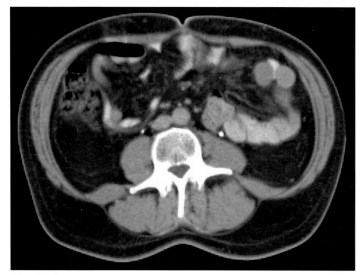

Fig. 88.1a

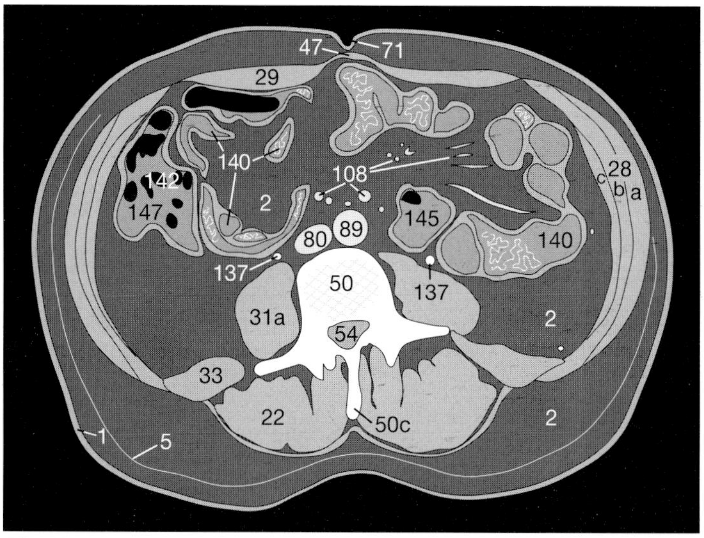

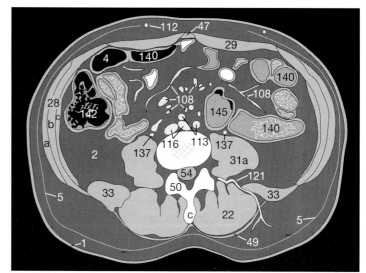

Fig. 88.1b

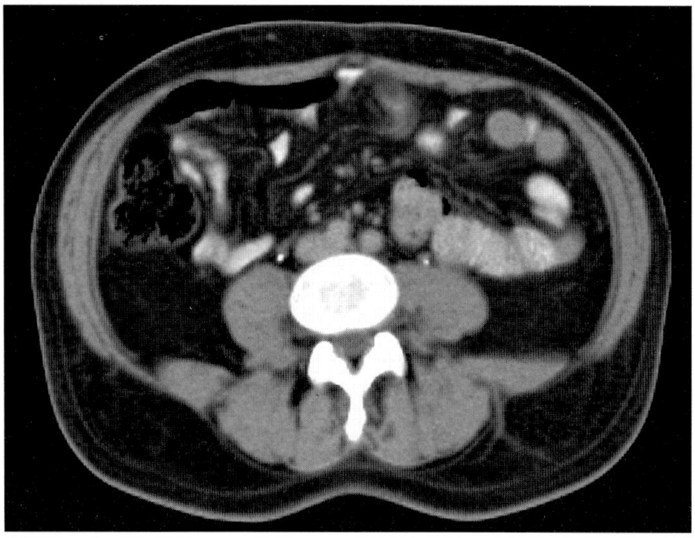

Fig. 88.2a

Fig. 88.2b

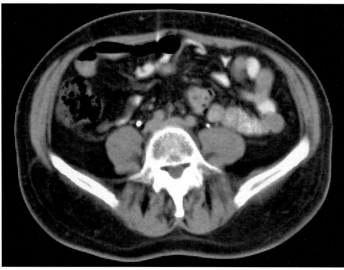

Fig. 88.3a

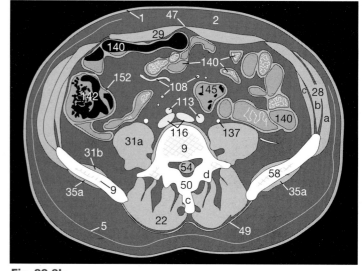

Fig. 88.3b

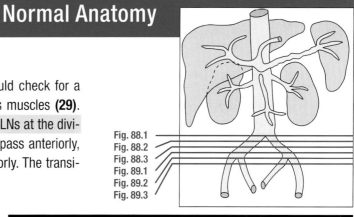

Fig. 88.1
Fig. 88.2
Fig. 88.3
Fig. 89.1
Fig. 89.2
Fig. 89.3

In order to exclude the presence of an abdominal hernia you should check for a normal width of the linea alba **(47)** between the rectus abdominis muscles **(29)**. More caudally **(Fig. 89.3)** there is a site of predilection for enlarged LNs at the division of the iliac vessels into external artery/vein **(115/118)**, which pass anteriorly, and internal artery/vein **(114/117)**, which are located more posteriorly. The transition from the lumbar spine **(50)** to the sacrum **(62)** lies at this level.

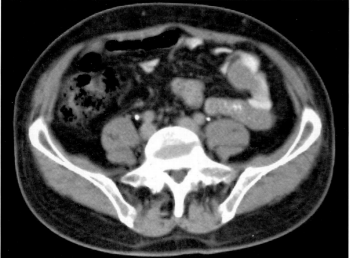

Fig. 89.1a

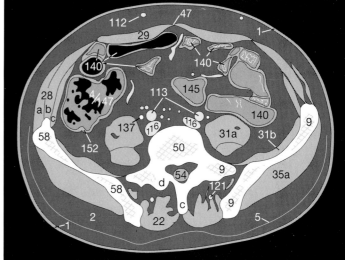

Fig. 89.1b

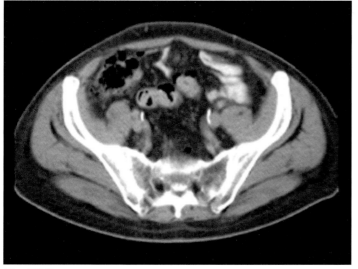

Fig. 89.2a

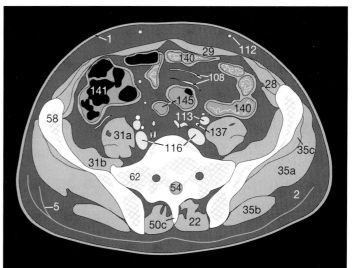

Fig. 89.2b

Fig. 89.3a

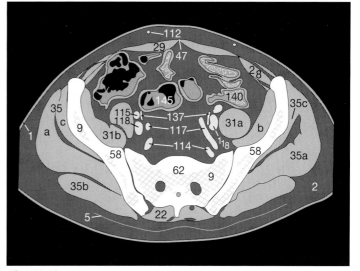

Fig. 89.3b

In the following images, the ureters **(137)** pass posteriorly to approach the lateral aspects of the base of the bladder **(138)**. Within the bladder, differences in the concentration of excreted CM in the urine can be recognized as fluid–fluid levels of different densities (**Figs. 90.3** and **91.1**). On the next page, a male pelvis is shown, demonstrating the prostate **(153)**, seminal vesicle **(154)**, spermatic cord **(155)**, and root of penis **(156)**. Note in particular the internal obturator muscles **(41a)** and the levator ani muscles **(42)** lateral to the anal canal **(146a)**; images of the female pelvis on pages 92/93 were not obtained as far caudally as in the male.

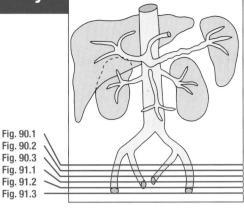

Fig. 90.1
Fig. 90.2
Fig. 90.3
Fig. 91.1
Fig. 91.2
Fig. 91.3

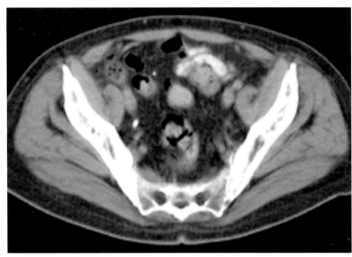

Fig. 90.1a

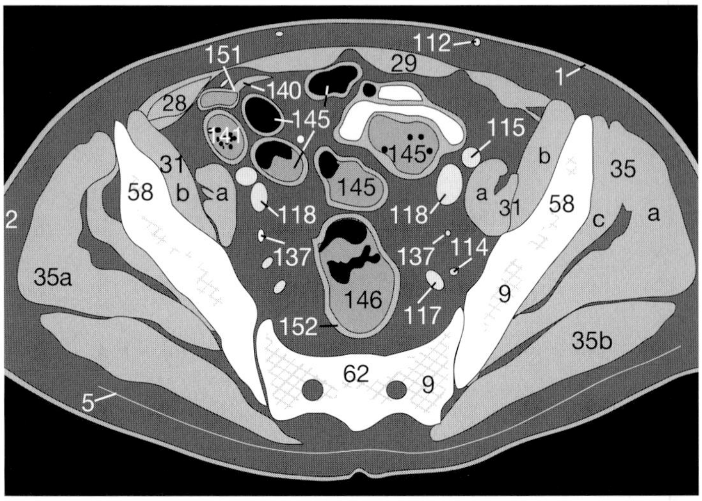

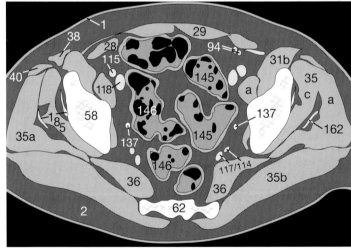

Fig. 90.1b

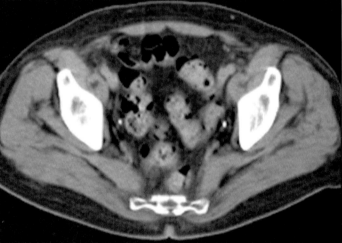

Fig. 90.2a

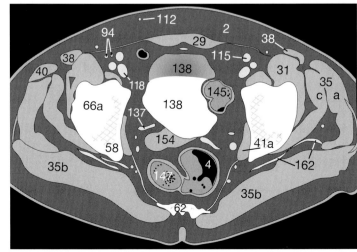

Fig. 90.2b

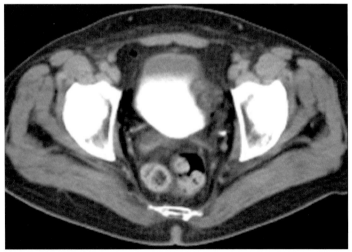

Fig. 90.3a

Fig. 90.3b

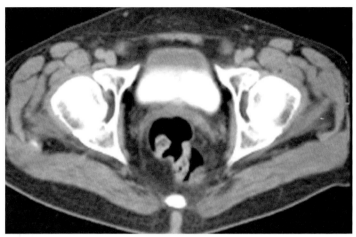

Fig. 91.1a

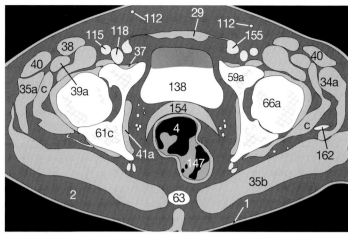

Fig. 91.1b

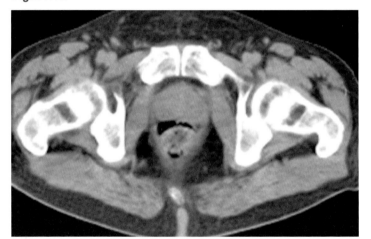

Fig. 91.2a

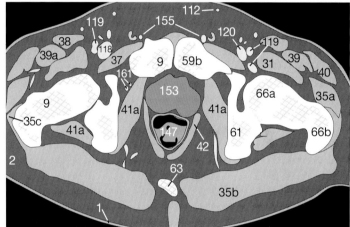

Fig. 91.2b

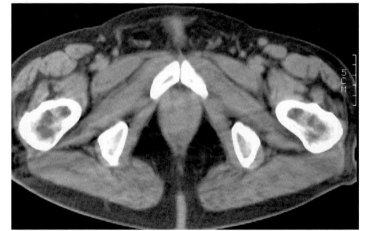

Fig. 91.3a

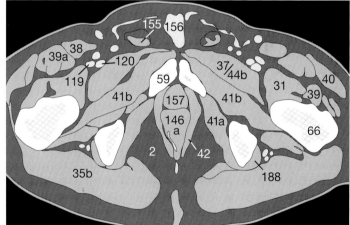

Fig. 91.3b

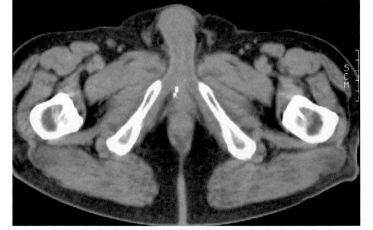

Fig. 91.4a

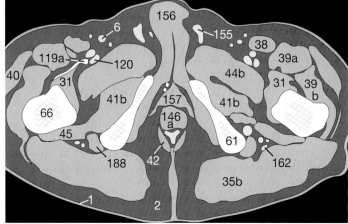

Fig. 91.4b

In the female pelvis the size and position of the uterus **(158)** relative to the urinary bladder can vary considerably from patient to patient. The uterus may lie cranial or lateral to the bladder (**Figs. 92.1–93.1**). The cervix and the vagina are situated between the bladder **(138)** and the rectum **(146)**, whereas the ovaries **(159)** lie more laterally. Depending on age and the phase of the menstrual cycle, ovarian follicles might be misinterpreted as cystic lesions (cf. p. 127).

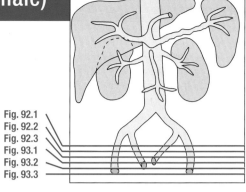

Fig. 92.1
Fig. 92.2
Fig. 92.3
Fig. 93.1
Fig. 93.2
Fig. 93.3

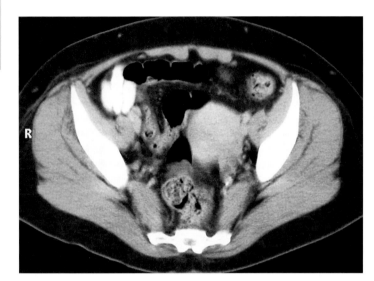

Fig. 92.1a

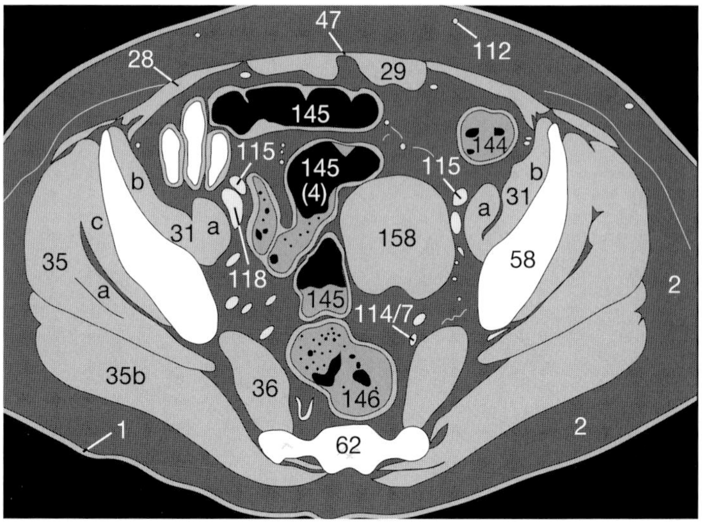

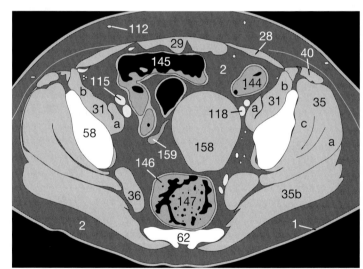

Fig. 92.1b

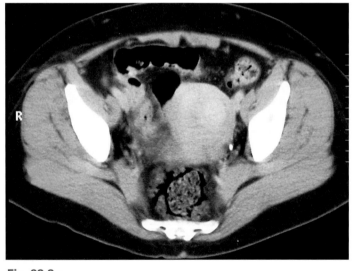

Fig. 92.2a

Fig. 92.2b

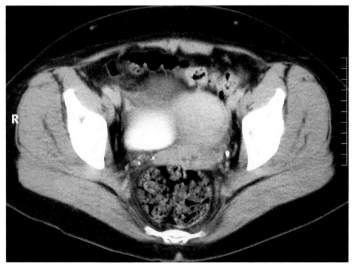

Fig. 92.3a

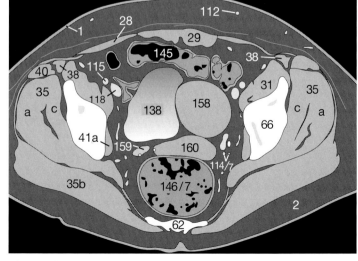

Fig. 92.3b

Free intra-abdominal fluid (ascites or hemorrhage) may occur in the rectouterine pouch between rectum and uterus, as well as in the vesicouterine space. In the inguinal region lymph nodes (6) can be up to 2 cm in diameter and be normal (**Figs. 93.2** and **93.3**). The size of normal abdominal lymph nodes does not usually exceed 1 cm. It is not possible to examine the hip joints on soft-tissue windows (**Fig. 93.3**); the heads of the femurs (66a) in the acetabular fossae (59/61) can best be analyzed on bone windows (not shown here). An assessment of bone windows completes the examination of the abdominal and pelvic images.

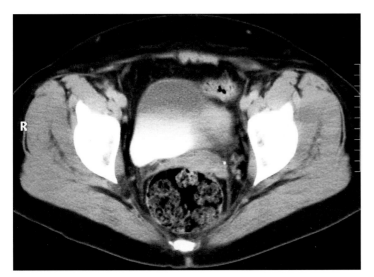

Fig. 93.1a

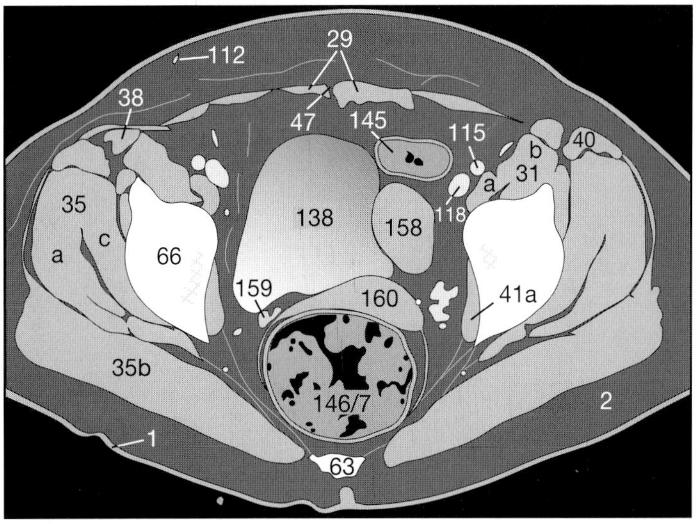

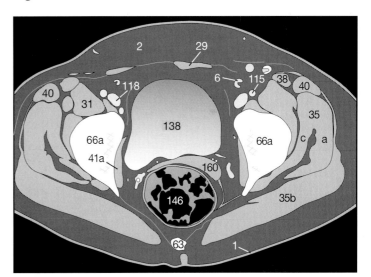

Fig. 93.1b

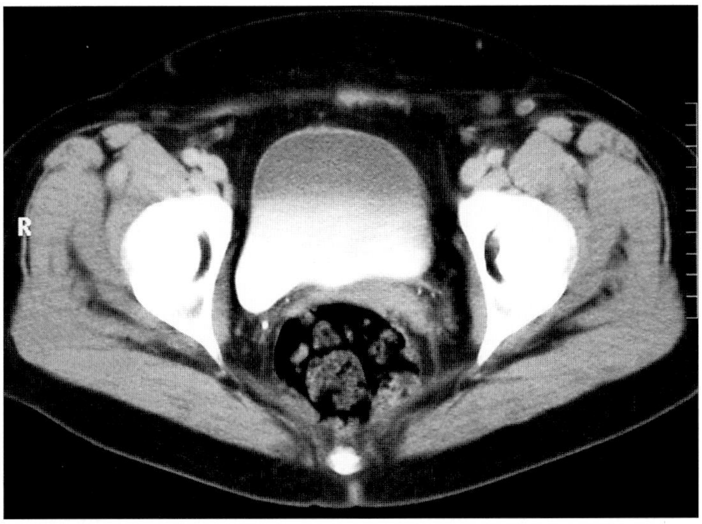

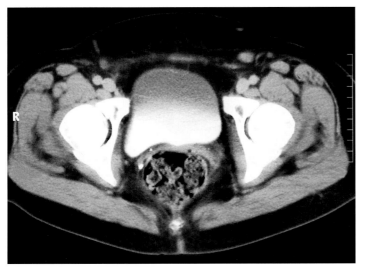

Fig. 93.2a

Fig. 93.2b

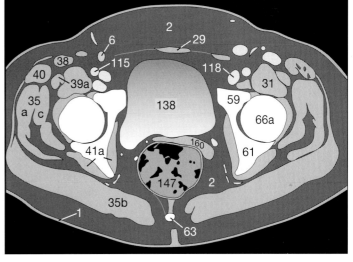

Fig. 93.3a

Fig. 93.3b

Segments of the Lung

It is especially important to be able to identify the segments of the lungs in CT images if bronchioscopy is planned for biopsy or to remove a foreign body. The right lung has 10 segments. In the left lung the apical and posterior upper lobe segments have a common bronchus and there is no 7th segment (paracardiac [medial basal] segment of the lower lobe).

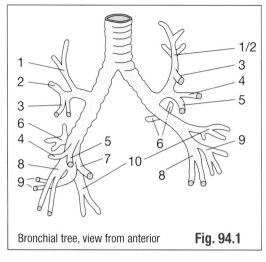

Bronchial tree, view from anterior **Fig. 94.1**

Upper lobe	1	apical
	2	posterior
	3	anterior
Middle lobe	4	lateral (superior lingula)
	5	medial (inferior lingula)
Lower lobe	6	superior/apical
	7	paracardiac/medial basal
	8	anterior basal
	9	lateral basal
	10	posterior basal

The parenchyma next to the interlobular fissures (——) appears avascular.

The borders of the segments (··········) are usually not visible in sections of normal thickness and can only be identified by the branches of the pulmonary veins (**96**) which pass along these borders.

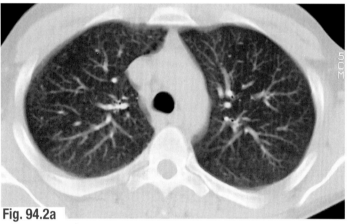

Fig. 94.2a

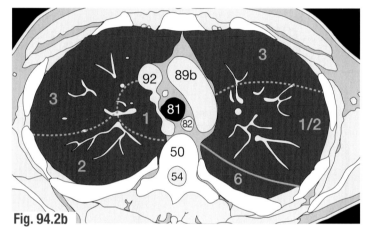

Fig. 94.2b

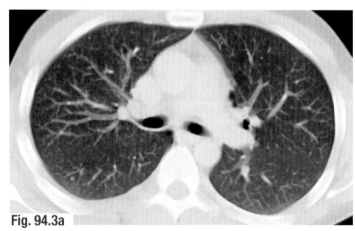

Fig. 94.3a

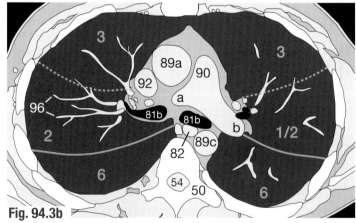

Fig. 94.3b

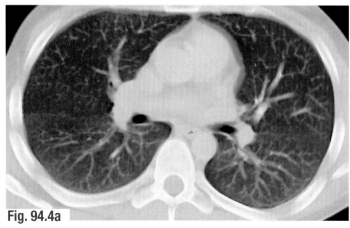

Fig. 94.4a

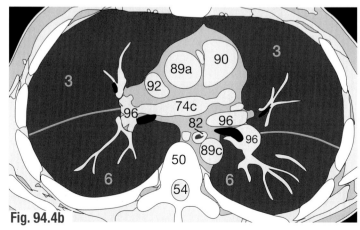

Fig. 94.4b

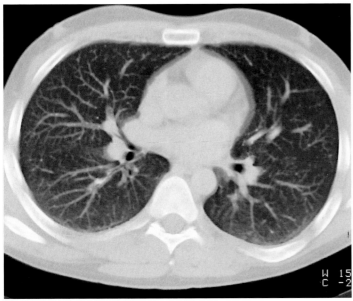

Fig. 95.1a

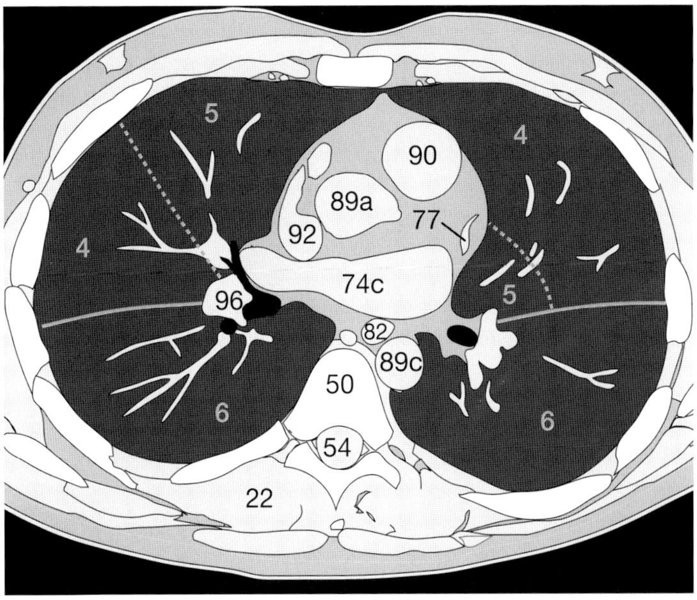

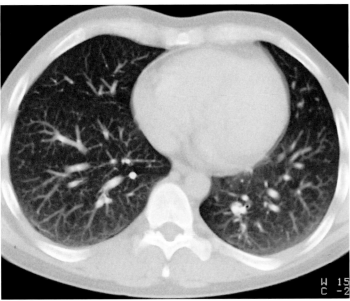

Fig. 95.1b

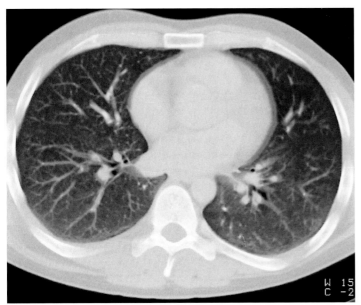

Fig. 95.2a

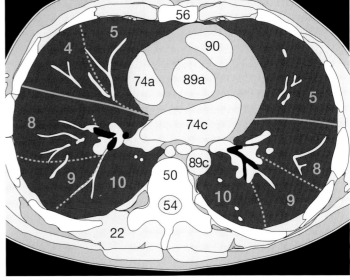

Fig. 95.2b

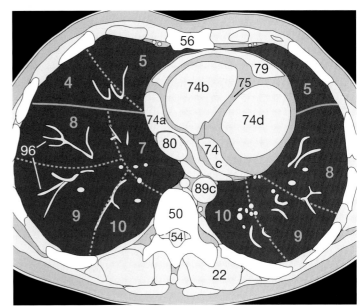

Fig. 95.3a

Fig. 95.3b

High-Resolution Technique

HRCT stands for *h*igh-*r*esolution *c*omputed *t*omography using thin sections and a high spatial resolution reconstruction algorithm. Even conventional CT scanners can acquire images of narrower d$_S$ than the standard 8–10 mm. The image acquisition parameters can be adjusted on the console to a thickness of 1–2 mm if necessary.

In the SCT technique, thinner sections can also be computed at a pitch factor of 1:1 after acquisition (see also p. 163). However, it is not usually worth reconstructing slices of less than 1 mm thickness because the low signal-to-noise ratio reduces image quality.

HRCT is therefore not the method of choice for routine chest examination because radiation dosage is much higher if more sections are acquired. Longer examination times and higher hard-copy film cost are also arguments against using HRCT. Only structures with naturally high levels of contrast such as areas surrounding bone will be well demonstrated.

High-Resolution Effects on Image Quality

Figure 96.1 shows a conventional scan of a pulmonary lesion **(7)** surrounded by a zone of edema or an infiltrate **(185)**. At a d$_S$ setting of 10 mm this zone closely resembles the poorly ventilated area at the back of the posterior lobe **(178)**.

HRCT distinguishes these areas of increased density more clearly **(Fig. 96.2)** because voxel averaging does not have any appreciable effect (see also p. 10).

The DD includes bronchial carcinoma, metastasis of breast cancer resulting in lymphangitis carcinomatosa, and atypical pneumonia.

These images show a rare complication after catheterization of the right heart. The catheter was positioned too peripherally and caused hemorrhage **(173)** into adjacent parts of the lung. Follow-up 3 weeks later showed complete recovery.

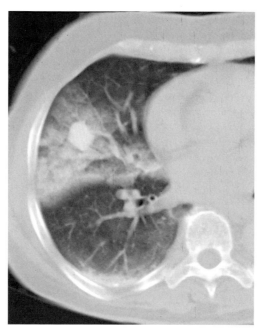

Fig. 96.1a

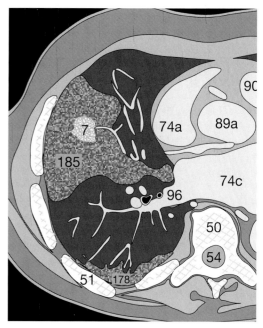

Fig. 96.1b

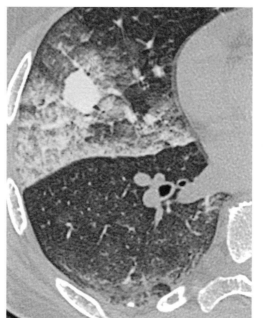

Fig. 96.2a

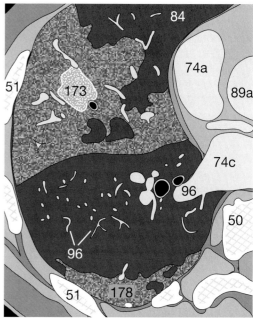

Fig. 96.2b

Indications

One of the many advantages of the HRCT technique is that older scar tissue can be distinguished from acute inflammation, for example in immune-suppressed patients or bone marrow recipients. Older scar tissue **(186)** is always well defined **(Fig. 97.1)**, whereas fresh infiltrates are surrounded by a zone of edematous tissue **(185)** as in **Figure 97.2**. HRCT is often the only method with which to determine whether chemotherapy should be continued in a lymphoma patient who is in the aplastic phase on therapy or whether chemotherapy must be discontinued because of fungal pneumonia. Fresh infiltrates **(178)** can sometimes be seen next to older scar tissue **(186)** **(Fig. 97.3)**.

Because the slices are extremely thin, the horizontal interlobular fissure (⋆) may appear as a bizarre ring or crescentic (**Figs. 97.1** and **97.2**).

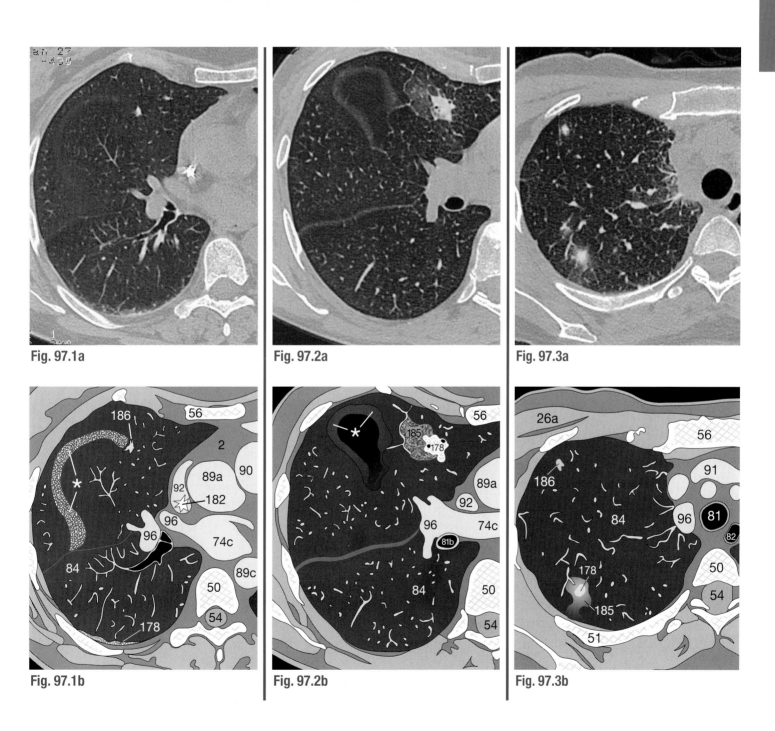

Fig. 97.1a

Fig. 97.2a

Fig. 97.3a

Fig. 97.1b

Fig. 97.2b

Fig. 97.3b

Minor areas of collapse, which are usually found close to the pleura posteriorly in the lung, must be differentiated from flat sections of fissures (**178** in **Fig. 97.1**). In doubtful cases, it may be helpful to repeat a scan in the prone position. Areas of collapse and poor ventilation may then disappear or be seen anteriorly. Pulmonary abnormalities due to an infiltrate or to a pneumoconiosis would be unchanged.

Among the many anatomic variations of the thorax, an atypical course of the azygos vein **(140)** is relatively common. It can pass from the posterior mediastinum through the right apical lobe to the superior vena cava **(92)**. It is located within a fold of the pleura and therefore separates the azygos lobe from the remainder of the right upper lobe. This variation is usually discovered incidentally on a conventional chest X-ray (↗ in **Fig. 98.1**) and has no clinical significance. **Figures 98.2** to **98.4** show the anomalous path of the vessel as it appears in CT images. Atypical positions or branching of the aortic arch **(89)** vessels are rarer. An example is the right subclavian artery, known as the "Arteria lusoria," which can resemble a lesion in the upper mediastinum.

Note that normal breast tissue, surrounded by fat **(2)**, may have very irregular contours (**72** in **Fig. 98.4**).

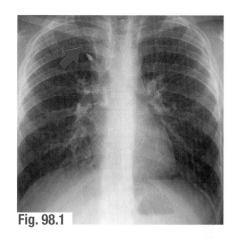

Fig. 98.1

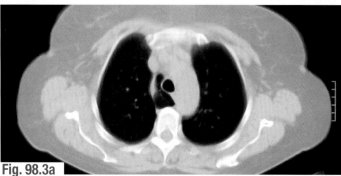

Fig. 98.2a

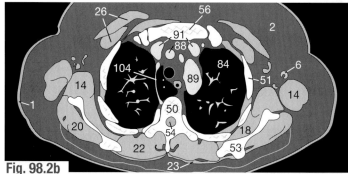

Fig. 98.2b

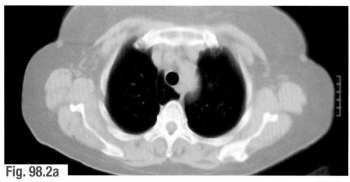

Fig. 98.3a

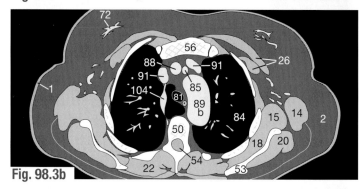

Fig. 98.3b

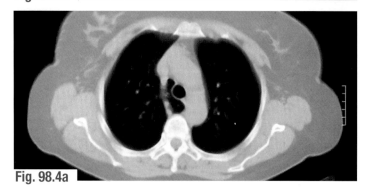

Fig. 98.4a

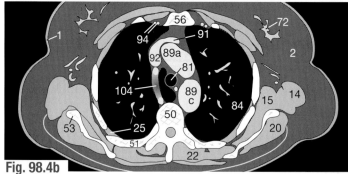

Fig. 98.4b

When using lung windows, you should not only look for solid round lesions and inflammatory infiltrates, but also recognize any thinning or even absence of lung vessels. However, attenuation of vessels is not always a sign of emphysema. Asymmetry in the bronchovascular pattern develops after a part of the lung has been resected. In the patient imaged in **Figure 98.5**, the left upper lobe had been removed and the remaining lung tissue has compensated and filled the entire left thoracic cavity (right half of the image). There are fewer lung vessels per unit volume and an ipsilateral shift of the mediastinum. These changes are accompanied by a slight elevation of the diaphragm. At the time of this follow-up CT, the patient was healthy and had neither emphysema nor recurrent tumor.

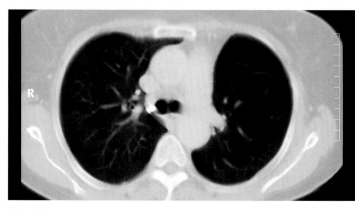

Fig. 98.5

According to the sequence in the checklist on page 72, one should now turn to soft-tissue windows in order to examine the soft tissues of the chest wall. Most abnormalities will be located in the axillae and in the female breast.

Alterations in Lymph Nodes

Normal axillary LNs (6) are usually oval and less than 1 cm in dimension. They often have a hypodense center or are horseshoe-shaped as in **Figure 99.1**, a feature known as the "hilum fat sign." The architecture of a normal LN is characterized by vessels entering the hilum, which contains hypodense fat. Many abnormal LNs have lost their normal contours and are rounder or irregular. Such LNs all appear solid and lack the hilum fat sign, as seen in those in the left axilla in **Figure 99.2**. For direct comparison, two lymph nodes on the other side in the same image are normal.

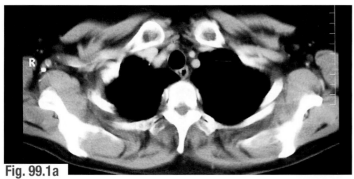

Fig. 99.1a

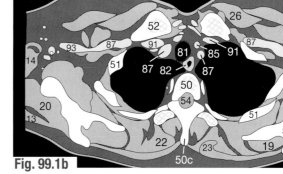

Fig. 99.1b

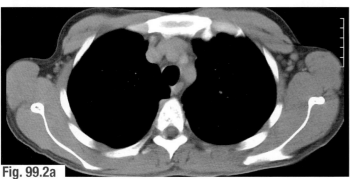

Fig. 99.2a

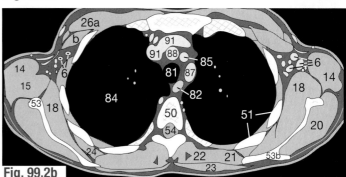

Fig. 99.2b

Larger metastatic LNs (7) are usually poorly defined and difficult to differentiate from surrounding fat (2). They often have central areas of necrosis (181), so that the differential diagnosis of an abscess with central liquefaction must be considered (Fig. 99.3). If axillary lymph node metastases have been treated operatively or with radiotherapy, the date and treatment should be noted on the referral sheet for follow-up CT. Postoperative healing processes and scarring (186) change the morphology of LNs (Fig. 99.4), so they resemble abnormal nodes (see above). Again the lack of clinical information makes diagnosis unnecessarily difficult for the radiologist.

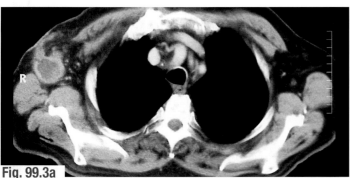

Fig. 99.3a

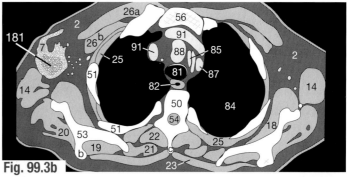

Fig. 99.3b

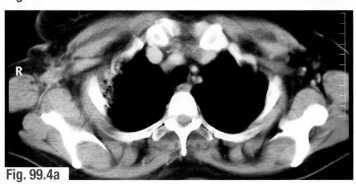

Fig. 99.4a

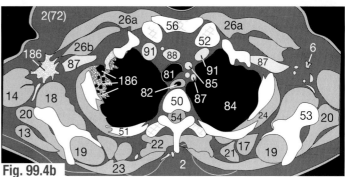

Fig. 99.4b

Breast

The normal parenchyma **(72)** of the female breast has very irregular contours and slender, finger-like extensions into the surrounding fat **(2)** (cf. **Fig. 98.4**). Bizarre shapes can often be seen **(Fig. 100.1)**. Advanced stages of breast cancer **(7)** have a solid, irregular appearance **(Fig. 100.1)**. The malignant tissue crosses the fascial planes or infiltrates the thoracic wall, depending on size. Baseline CT after mastectomy **(Fig. 100.2)** should help in the early identification of recurrent tumor. The diagnosis of recurrent tumor is made more difficult by fibrosis after radiation, postoperative scar tissue, and the absence of surrounding fat. Special attention must therefore be paid to the regional LNs (cf. p. 99) and the bones, so that metastases **(7)** in the vertebrae **(50)** **(Fig. 100.2)** are not overlooked. The bone window must be examined in such cases.

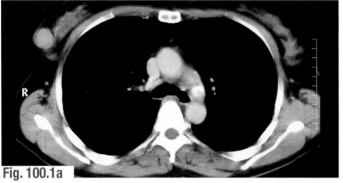

Fig. 100.1a

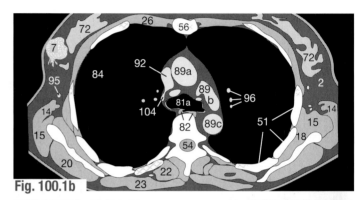

Fig. 100.1b

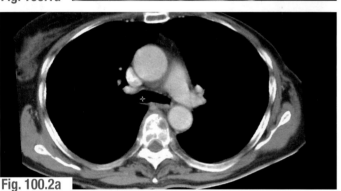

Fig. 100.2a

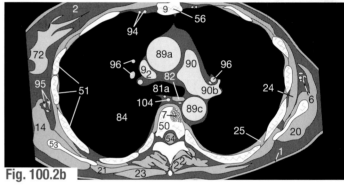

Fig. 100.2b

Thoracic Skeleton

Osteolysis within the thoracic skeleton is not uncommon and is usually due to either metastases or a plasma cell tumor. In **Figure 100.3** a metastasis **(7)** from a thyroid carcinoma has destroyed part of the left clavicle **(52)**. Osteolysis can, however, also be caused by an enchondroma or an eosinophilic granuloma, for example of a rib. In addition to destructive processes (cf. **Fig. 20.3**), degenerative processes involving sclerosis and osteophyte formation of bone must be differentiated from osteosclerotic metastases which are typical of, for example, prostate carcinoma (cf. p. 139).

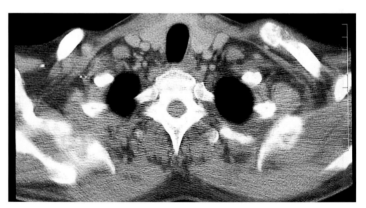

Fig. 100.3a

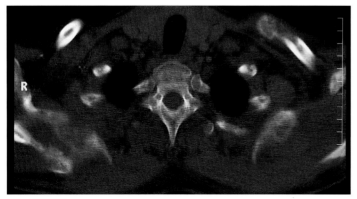

Fig. 100.3b

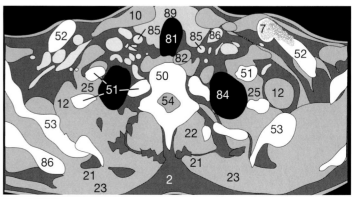

Fig. 100.3c

Before being able to detect lesions and lymphadenopathy, you must know the normal anatomy. If you are a preclinical student, you should firstly study normal sectional anatomy. It is in your own interests to work through the following pages only when you are sufficiently familiar with the previous chapters.

Tumors

A benign increase in fat **(2)** due to cortisone therapy is occasionally observed in the anterior mediastinum **(Fig. 101.1)**. In doubtful cases, densitometry is helpful in the DD (cf. p. 11). In this example, the average density within the region of interest (ROI), which is positioned in possible fatty tissue, is −89.3 HU with a standard deviation of about 20 HU (cf. **Table 12.1**). As a rule, the size of an ROI in cm² is also provided **(Fig. 101.1)**. The DD of such a mass would include retrosternal goiter and thymoma.

In children and young adults the density of the thymus is about +45 HU. As a result of involution, the density of the organ decreases with age from the third decade onward until it has dropped to the density typical of fat (−90 HU). The left lobe of the thymus is often larger than the right and can reach the aortopulmonary window. A lobe should not be thicker than 1.3 cm in adults; up to the age of 20, 1.8 cm is considered normal.

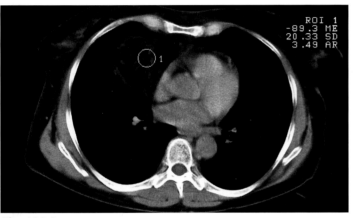

Fig. 101.1a

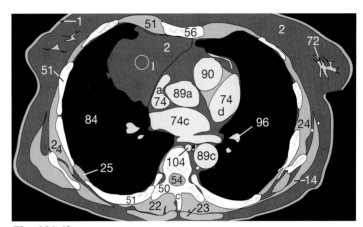

Fig. 101.1b

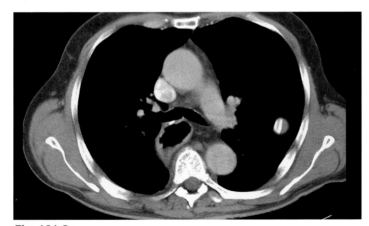

Fig. 101.2a

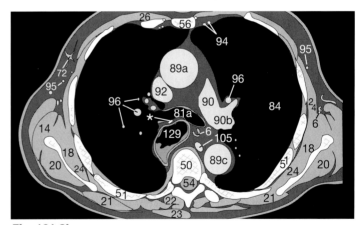

Fig. 101.2b

Malignant thickening of the walls of the esophagus must be differentiated from gastric conduits following esophageal surgery **(Fig. 101.2)**. Possible enlargement of LNs **(6)** next to the stomach **(129)** must be excluded by follow-up CTs. Occasionally postoperative metal clips cause artifacts (✱) which make assessment of the mediastinum more difficult. Following esophageal resection, parts of the colon (➡) may become drawn up into the anterior mediastinum **(Fig. 101.3)**. Comparison with adjacent sections quickly shows that this structure is not an emphysematous bulla, but is a tubular organ containing a lumen.

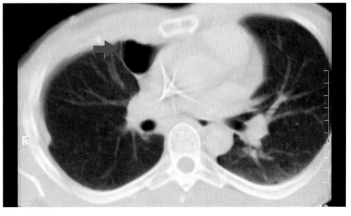

Fig. 101.3

Enlarged Lymph Nodes

Normal LNs are often found at the level of the aortopulmonary window. They are mainly oval or irregular, less than 10 mm across [19] and sharply delineated from mediastinal fat **(2)**. LNs **(6)** in this area are not usually considered suspicious until they exceed 1.5 cm in diameter. The demonstration of a "hilum fat sign" (cf. p. 99) is not obligatory, but does suggest a benign nature **(Fig. 102.1)**.

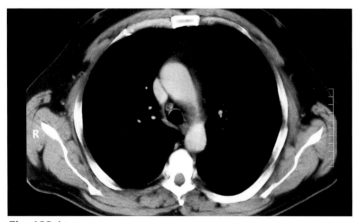

Fig. 102.1a

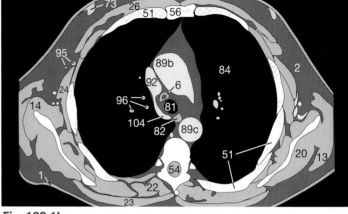

Fig. 102.1b

If more than three LNs are seen in the aortopulmonary window or if a single LN is abnormally enlarged, the DD includes not only a metastasis from a bronchial carcinoma, but also a lymphoma **(Fig. 102.2)**.

Enlarged mediastinal, and especially hilar, LNs are also characteristic of sarcoidosis (Boeck's disease) **(6 in Fig. 102.3)**. In **Figure 102.2** there are intrapulmonary metastases **(7)** as well. Did you notice them? Other sites of predilection for abnormal LNs are anterior to the aortic arch, beneath the bifurcation of the trachea (subcarinal), and the para-aortic and retrocrural regions.

Normal size (diameter) of LNs [19, 41]:

• anterior mediastinum	< 6 mm
• aortopulmonary window	< 15 mm
• hilar	< 10 mm
• subcarinal	< 10 mm
• para-aortic	< 7 mm

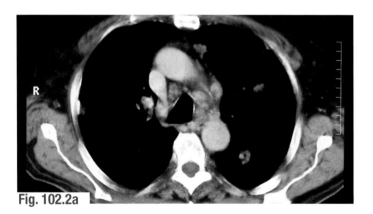

Fig. 102.2a

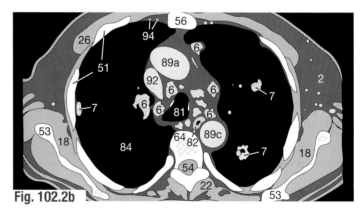

Fig. 102.2b

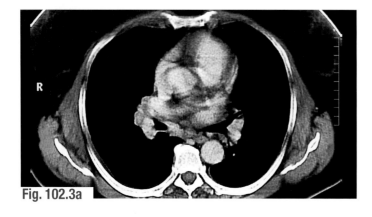

Fig. 102.3a

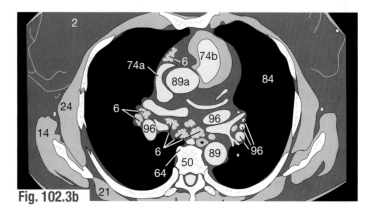

Fig. 102.3b

Vascular Pathologies

Inflow phenomena of CM injected through an arm vein (cf. p. 19) and anomalous vessels (cf. p. 98) in the mediastinum have already been discussed. Incompletely mixed CM must be distinguished from a possible thrombus (173) in the lumen of the brachiocephalic vein (91). Such a thrombus can adhere to a central venous catheter (182 in Fig. 103.1).

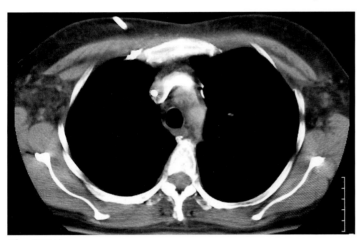

Fig. 103.1a

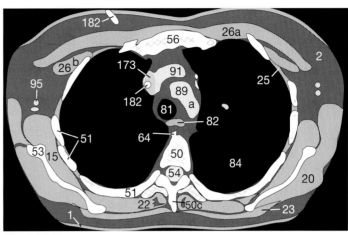

Fig. 103.1b

Atherosclerotic plaques (174) in the aorta (89) are often accompanied by thrombotic deposits (173 in Fig. 103.3). They promote aortic elongation and dilation and can ultimately lead to an aneurysm (171). Dilation of the thoracic aorta is considered to be an aneurysm if the lumen is wider than 4 cm. Recording the measurements of distances and sizes (Fig. 103.2) makes it easier to assess any progressive dilation in follow-up CTs. It is important to check for any involvement of the branches of the great vessels or for the presence of a dissection flap (172 in Fig. 103.4). Three types of dissection can be diagnosed according to the extent of the dissection flap (see de Bakey [20]).

A true aneurysm with a diameter of more than 6 cm, with a more saccular than fusiform shape or with an eccentric lumen, has a higher incidence of rupture. The consequences of rupture include a mediastinal hematoma, a hemothorax, or pericardial tamponade.

Dissecting Aneurysms of the Aorta
(according to de Bakey [20])

Type I (approx. 50%)
    Ascending aorta; may extend to abdominal bifurcation

Type II (approx. 15%)
    Only ascending aorta, extending to brachiocephalic trunk

Type III (approx. 25%)
    Torn intima; distal to left subclavian artery

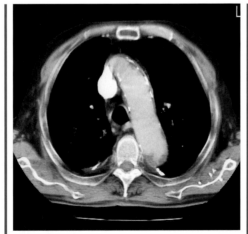

Fig. 103.3a

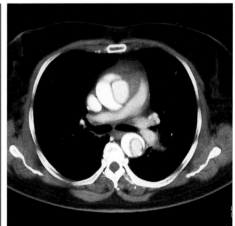

Fig. 103.4a

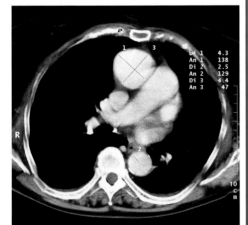

Fig. 103.2

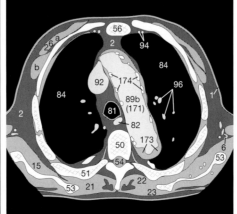

Fig. 103.3b

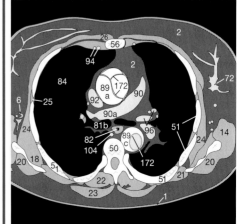

Fig. 103.4b

Pulmonary Embolism

If a large embolus has detached from a thrombus in a deep vein of the leg, it will be visible as a hypodense area (➘) within the involved pulmonary artery on contrast-enhanced images (Fig. 104.1). After large pulmonary emboli, the affected segments or lobes (➘) usually become poorly ventilated and atelectasis occurs. The pulmonary vessels become attenuated, which can be demonstrated in conventional x-rays.

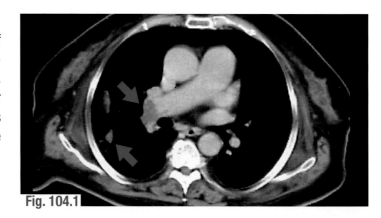
Fig. 104.1

Heart

You have already familiarized yourself with the normal anatomy of the heart on pages 77 to 79. Dilation resulting from valvular incompetence or from cardiomyopathies, as well as intracardiac filling defects can be recognized in CT images. If CM has been injected, it is possible to detect atrial thrombus or a thrombosed ventricular aneurysm. The image in **Figure 104.2** illustrates a case of global cardiac failure with markedly dilated atria (✱✱) and incidental thoracic vertebral degenerative osteophytes(➡).

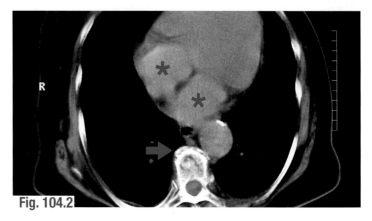
Fig. 104.2

Pericardial effusions may occur with viral infections, uremia, the collagen vascular diseases, a heart attack, or tuberculosis, among other causes. A pericardial effusion **(8)** appears as a broad rim of low-density fluid (between 10 and 40 HU) surrounding the heart **(Fig. 104.3)**. Only fresh blood would have a higher level of density. Massive effusions as seen in **Figure 104.3** not only compress the adjacent lungs **(178)**, but also compromise heart function.

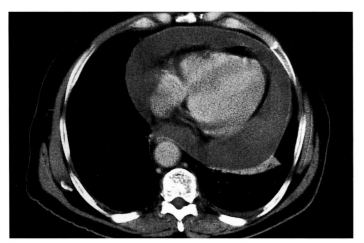
Fig. 104.3a

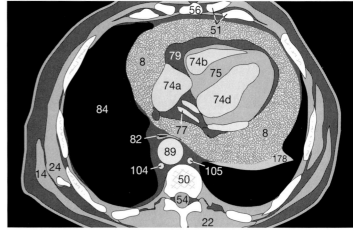
Fig. 104.3b

Effusions may lead to pericardial fibrosis or calcification (➘ ➚), which in turn causes constrictive pericarditis (Fig. 104.4). Note that in such cases the vena cava, the azygos vein, or even the atria may be markedly dilated as a sign of cardiac insufficiency.

Atherosclerosis of the coronary arteries causes calcification that is well demonstrated by thin, hyperdense lines in the epicardial fat. At present, however, a complete assessment of the degree of stenosis requires angiography.

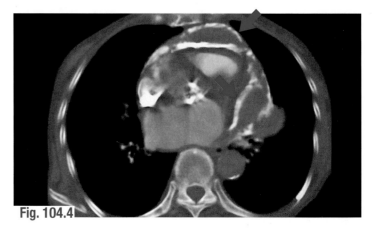
Fig. 104.4

Focal Intrapulmonary Lesions

When multiple lung metastases are far advanced, the lesions can even be recognized in the topogram (**Fig. 105.1a**). Depending upon the age and vascularization of the metastases, they appear as spherical nodules of varying sizes (**Fig. 105.1b**). The more irregular the contours of the lesions (for example, stellate or spicu- lated), the more likely they are to be malignant. If, however, they are solitary and have central calcification (like a popcorn), or peripheral calcification, the lesions are most likely to be a benign hamartoma or granuloma.

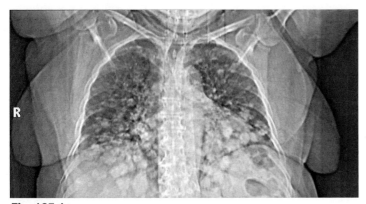

Fig. 105.1a

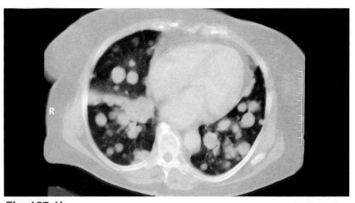

Fig. 105.1b

Pulmonary metastases are not visible in conventional X-rays unless they are larger than 5 or 6 mm in diameter. In CT images, however, they can be detected at 1 to 2 mm in diameter. If metastases are located in the periphery, it is easy to differentiate them from blood vessels cut in cross-section. Small metastases located close to the hilum are much more difficult to distinguish from vessels. In such cases the detailed analysis of high-resolution scans (HRCT) may be the best method.

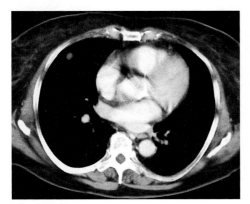

Fig. 105.2a

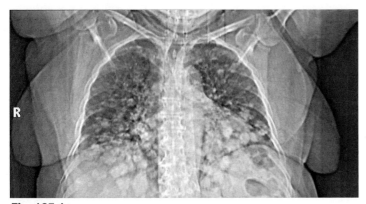

Fig. 105.2b

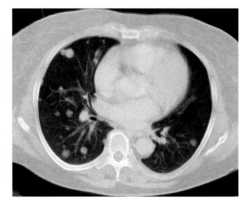

Fig. 105.2c

The correct choice of image display (window) is essential: Small focal lesions (**7**) of the lung (**84**) do not appear on soft-tissue windows (**Fig. 105.2a**) or may be mistaken for normal vessels (**96**). Lung windows (**Fig. 105.2c**) should always be used for examining lung parenchyma. In the case below (**Fig. 105.3a**), the multiple small metastases (**7**) close to the pleura would have been overlooked if lung windows had not been used (**Fig. 105.3c**). These examples demonstrate the importance of viewing each image on long and soft-tissue windows.

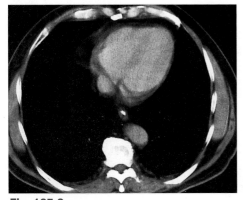

Fig. 105.3a

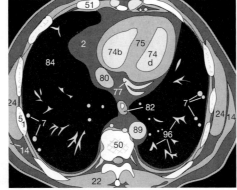

Fig. 105.3b

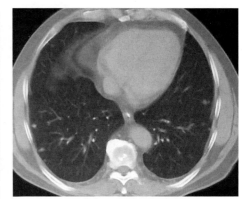

Fig. 105.3c

As a result of changes in the behavior of smokers, the incidence of bronchial carcinomas (BC), especially among women and young people, has increased. In addition to the histologic diagnosis and grading of carcinoma, the location of the lesion is an important prognostic factor: a BC of considerable size **(7)** in the periphery of the lung **(Fig. 106.1)** will almost certainly be visible on a con-

ventional chest X-ray. More advanced BCs located centrally are usually not operable and may obstruct the bronchial lumen resulting in distal collapse **(178)**. **Figure 106.2** illustrates an advanced case in which the tumor has areas of central necrosis **(181)** and the lung is surrounded by a pleural effusion **(8)**.

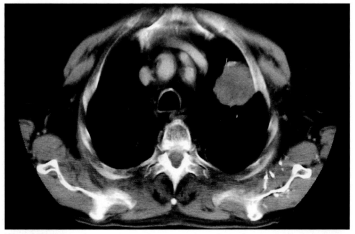

Fig. 106.1a

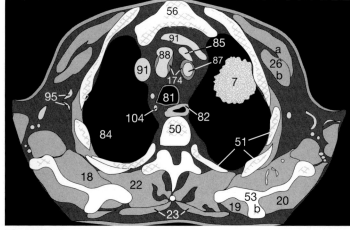

Fig. 106.1b

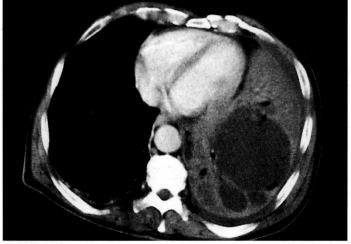

Fig. 106.2a

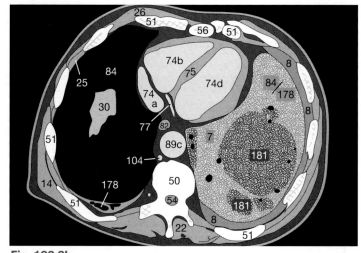

Fig. 106.2b

Lymphangitis carcinomatosa **(7** in **Fig. 106.3)** spreads from the hilum or the visceral pleura into the interstitial tissue of the lung by way of the lymphatic vessels. Obstruction of these vessels by cancer cells leads to lymphatic congestion **(185)**. At first the upper lobes remain clear, but as the disease progresses these also become infiltrated. The larger lymphatics and LNs gradually become infiltrated by metastatic disease.

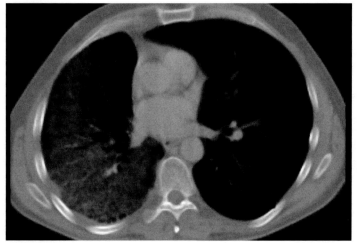

Fig. 106.3a

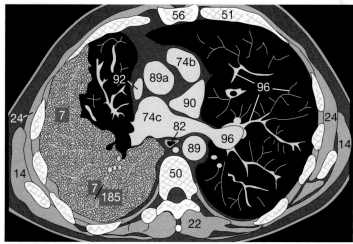

Fig. 106.3b

The changes of sarcoidosis (Boeck's disease) must be differentiated from multiple metastases in the lung: epithelial granulomas usually infiltrate the hilar lymph nodes **(6)** bilaterally **(Fig. 107.1)** and then spread within the perivascular tissue and along the lymphatics into the periphery of the lung. Multiple small pulmonary nodules and various degrees of interstitial fibrosis may be present. Large granulomas **(7)** as seen in **figure 107.2** may resemble intrapulmonary metastases.

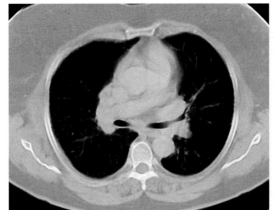

Fig. 107.1a

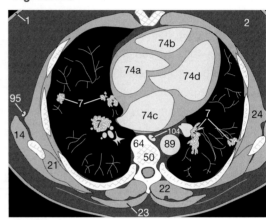

Fig. 107.1b

Fig. 107.2a

Fig. 107.2b

If a larger mass cavitates **(181)**, the DD will include, for example, a bronchial carcinoma with central necrosis or cavitary tuberculosis. **Figure 107.3** illustrates the latter in an atypical location in an HIV+, immune-compromised patient. Note also the emphysematous changes in the tissue at the periphery of the lesion **(176)**.

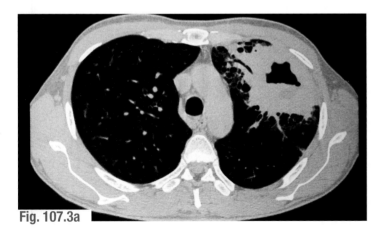

Fig. 107.3a

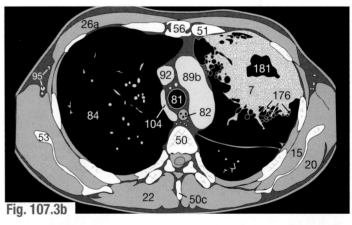

Fig. 107.3b

Superinfection with Aspergillus may occur within a pre-existing cavity in immune-compromised patients. The spores of A. fumigatus are common in plant material and soil. Often the cavity is not completely filled with the aspergillus ball so that a small crescent of air can be recognized (↘ in **Fig. 107.4**). Aspergillosis may also lead to allergic bronchial asthma or provoke exogenous, allergic alveolitis.

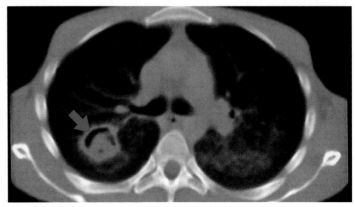

Fig. 107.4

Pleura

Massive pleural effusions **(8)**, as seen in the case illustrated in **Figure 108.1**, compress the lung **(84)** and may cause large areas of atelectasis **(178)** affecting individual segments or even an entire lobe. Effusions appear as collections of homogeneous fluid of near-water density within the pleural spaces. Effusions usually accompany infections, lung congestion due to right heart failure, as well as venous congestion due to mesothelioma and peripheral bronchial carcinoma. Pleural drainage by the insertion of a catheter **(182)** is indicated if atelectasis **(178)** affects large portions of the lung (**Fig. 108.2**). In the case shown in **Figure 108.2**, the drainage tube was blocked by fibrin-rich fluid. The lung can only be re-inflated if the fibrin clot is cleared or the catheter is replaced.

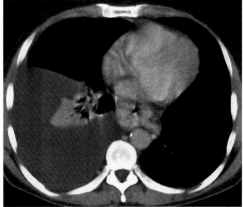

Fig. 108.1a

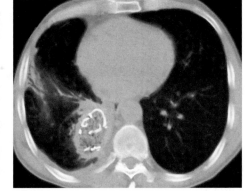

Fig. 108.1b

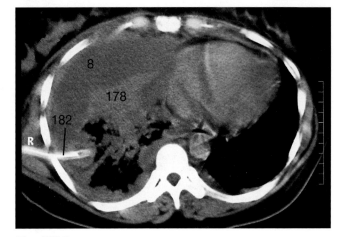

Fig. 108.2

Foreign bodies are rarely found in the pleural spaces (**166** in **Fig. 108.3**), but must be considered after thoracotomy (chest surgery). Images on lung windows (**Fig. 108.3c**) clearly show the inflammation and collapse **(178)** surrounding a lost swab.

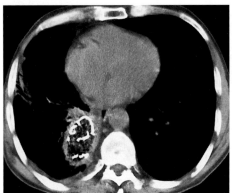

Fig. 108.3a

Fig. 108.3b

Fig. 108.3c

Asbestos-Related Lung Disease

Asbestos-related lung disease has a fine reticulonodular pattern of increased densities scattered throughout the lung tissue, especially at interlobular septa (⬆ and ⬈ in **Fig. 108.4**). Typical pathologic features in the pleura are thickening and plaques (**186** in **Fig. 108.4**). Fibrosis and scar emphysema appear in later stages of the disease. The spindle-shaped or more triangular areas of increased attenuation are often difficult to distinguish from those characteristic of bronchial carcinomas.

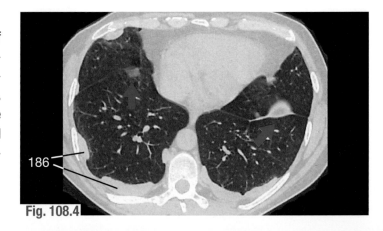

Fig. 108.4

Silicosis

Multiple, well-defined nodules appear in the interstitial connective tissue in response to phagocytosed particles of silica. The upper lobes of the lung are most commonly affected. Signs of fibrosis, which may progress to a honeycomb pattern, can best–and at earlier stages–be detected with HRCT (using 2-mm rather than 10-mm slice thickness; **Fig. 109.1**). The finer, smaller nodules can be found scattered throughout the lung; larger opacities, which may cavitate, are located within areas of denser fibrosis (↗ in **Fig. 109.2**). Enlarged mediastinal or hilar lymph nodes often develop an eggshell pattern of calcification. As the disease progresses, fibrosis and scar emphysema increase (← in **Fig. 109.1**).

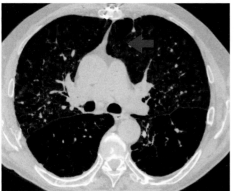

Fig. 109.1

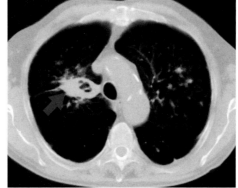

Fig. 109.2

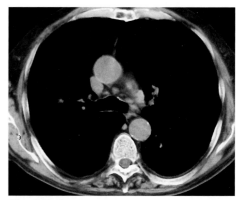

Fig. 109.3

Emphysema

Progressive emphysema with accompanying bullae (**176** in **Fig. 109.4b**) or bronchiectasis with associated inflammatory infiltrates (**178** in **Fig. 109.5b**) are not visible on soft-tissue window images in the early stages. These infiltrates are more easily seen and detected sooner on thin section images using lung windows [25–27].

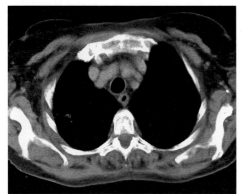

Fig. 109.4a

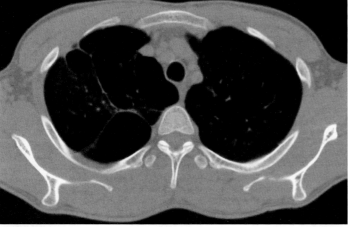

Fig. 109.4b

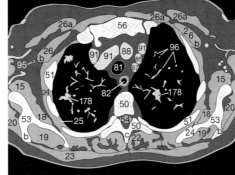

Fig. 109.5a

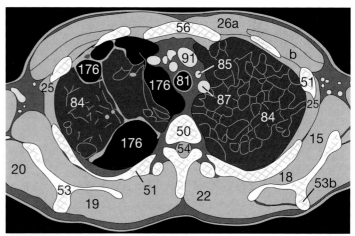

Fig. 109.5b

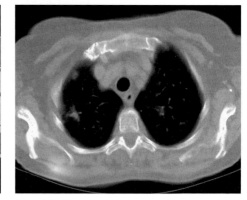

Fig. 109.5c

The pathogenesis of interstitial fibrosis of the lung **(Fig. 110.1)** cannot always be established and is referred to as idiopathic pulmonary fibrosis. This is particularly true when it affects middle-aged women. The pattern of fibrosis resembles that illustrated on the previous pages with the exception that emphysematous changes typically begin in subpleural regions. Fibrosis of the lung can accompany any of the collagen vascular diseases in the advanced stages and lead to similar morphologic changes, for example in scleroderma **(Fig. 110.2)** or polyarteritis nodosa **(Fig. 110.3)**.

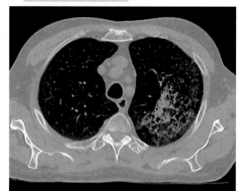

Fig. 110.1

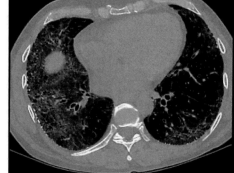

Fig. 110.2

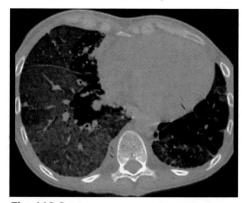

Fig. 110.3

Test Yourself!

You should try to answer all the questions on this and the following page before turning to the back of the book for the answers so as not to spoil the fun of tackling each one.

Exercise 20:
Do you recognize any abnormalities in **Figure 110.4** or is it a scan of normal anatomy? Discuss your DD.

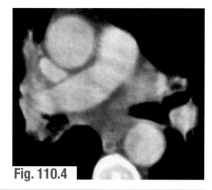

Fig. 110.4

Exercise 21:
How would you interpret the dense area in the left lung in **Figure 110.5**? Discuss your DD and make a list of additional information that you need and the steps necessary in order to be certain about the lesion.

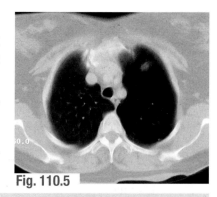

Fig. 110.5

Exercise 22:
A 62-year-old patient presented with intense back pain and was examined by CT. What is your diagnosis of the changes seen in **Figure 110.6**? Can you classify the type of change and the degree of severity?

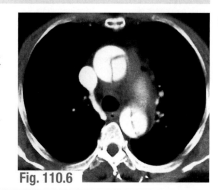

Fig. 110.6

Exercise 23: Describe in detail the pathologic changes visible in **Figure 110.7** and the steps in your DD.

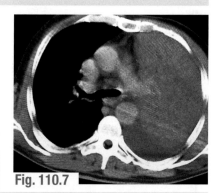

Fig. 110.7

Exercise 24:
What further diagnostic procedures would you recommend for the case illustrated in **Figure 111.1**? What do you suspect the lesion to be? What other changes do you recognize?

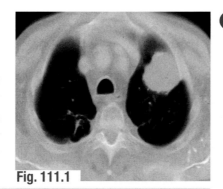

Fig. 111.1

Exercise 25:
Detecting even minute changes may be decisive in order to arrive at the correct diagnosis. What do you see in **Figure 111.2**?

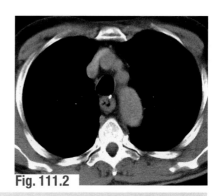

Fig. 111.2

Exercise 26:
A patient in her 26th week of pregnancy complained of shortness of breath. Her physician initially thought it was because of a high diaphragm. Two weeks later she was examined by CT. Make careful note of all abnormal changes you see in **Figure 111.3** and the steps in your DD.

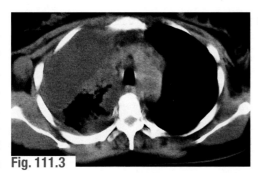

Fig. 111.3

Exercise 27:
A 56-year-old woman with a history of smoking presented with unintended weight loss and severe attacks of coughing which had already lasted for 3 months. She had no previous illnesses. Does **Figure 111.4** illustrate normal anatomy, a normal variant, or an abnormality?

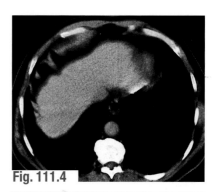

Fig. 111.4

Exercise 28: Do **Figures 111.5a** and **111.5b** illustrate normal anatomy, an anomaly, or a lymphoma? Discuss your opinion.

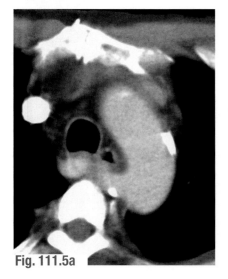

Fig. 111.5a

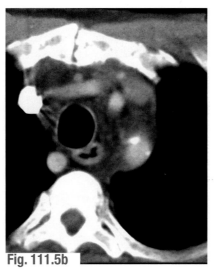

Fig. 111.5b

Anatomic Variations

For the beginner it is important to be familiar with the most common anatomic variations which may lead to misinterpretations of CT images. In some patients the contours of the right lobe of the liver **(122)** may appear scalloped by impressions of the diaphragm **(30)** which could be mistaken for liver lesions **(Fig. 112.1)**. The walls of an empty stomach (129) are thick and may suggest a malignant lesion **(129a)**.

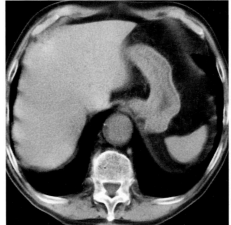

Fig. 112.1a

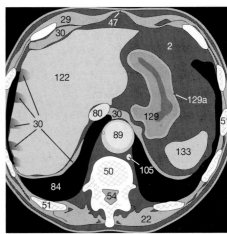

Fig. 112.1b

Ultrasound may mistake an anomalous left renal vein **(111)** for a retro-aortic LN. Usually the left renal vein passes between the SMA **(106)** and the aorta **(89)**. However, the vein may be retro-aortic and pass between the aorta and the spinal column **(50)** to the inferior vena cava **(80)** **(Figs. 112.2–112.4)**. Duplication of the left renal vein with preaortic and retroaortic components can also occur.

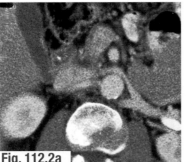

Fig. 112.2a

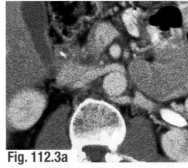

Fig. 112.3a

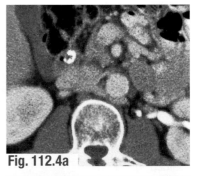

Fig. 112.4a

Fig. 112.2b

Fig. 112.3b

Fig. 112.4b

Characteristic Partial Volume Effects

If the wall of one organ indents that of another, cross-sectional images will make it look as if one organ were within the other. For example, the sigmoid colon **(145)** may appear "within" the urinary bladder **(138)** **(Fig. 112.5a)**. By comparing adjacent sections **(Figs. 112.5a** and **c)** it is easy to recognize that only parts of both organs have been imaged. In a similar manner, the right colic flexure **(142)** may appear to be "within" the gallbladder **(126)** **(Fig. 112.6)**.

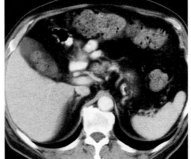

Fig. 112.6a

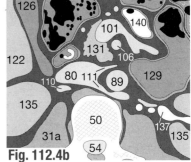

Fig. 112.6b

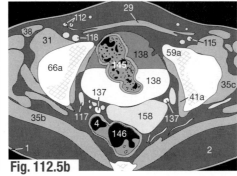

Fig. 112.5a

Fig. 112.5b

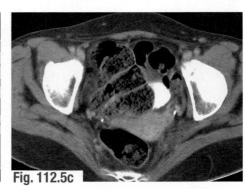

Fig. 112.5c

Lymph Node Hyperplasia

Pathologic lesions of the abdominal wall occur most frequently in the inguinal region. Lymph node hyperplasia with nodes up to 2 cm in dimension should not be considered abnormal. Large conglomerate masses of LNs (⬅) are found in non-Hodgkin's lymphoma (Fig. 113.1) and less frequently in Hodgkin's disease. An inguinal hematoma (173) caused by hemorrhage from a femoral artery puncture site after coronary angiography should be considered (Fig. 113.2) in the DD.

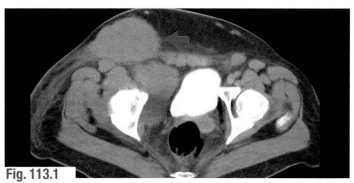

Fig. 113.1

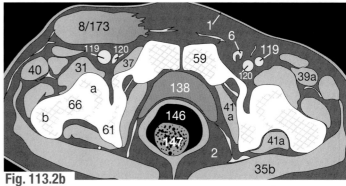

Fig. 113.2b

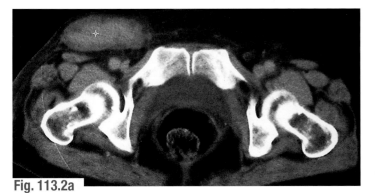

Fig. 113.2a

Abscesses

Intramuscular injection sites in the gluteal region resulting in subcutaneous fat (2) necrosis or postinflammatory residue (➡) typically are well defined, hyperdense, partially calcified lesions (Fig. 113.3). An abscess may spread from the gluteal muscles to the pelvis through the ischiorectal fossa. After diffuse infiltration (178) of the gluteal muscles (35) with surrounding edema (185 in Fig. 113.4), liquefaction (181) may occur and, depending on the localization and size, the abscess can involve the sciatic nerve (Fig. 113.5)

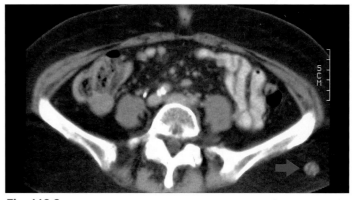

Fig. 113.3

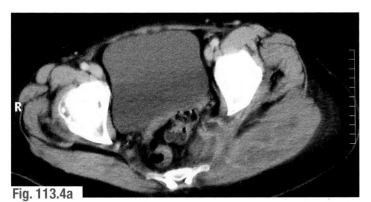

Fig. 113.4a

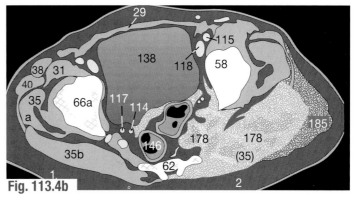

Fig. 113.4b

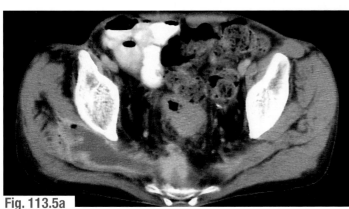

Fig. 113.5a

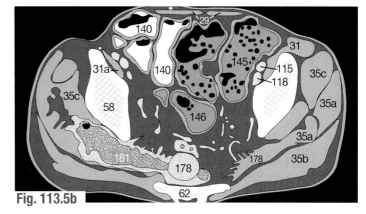

Fig. 113.5b

The CT in **Figure 114.1** shows subcutaneous lesions, resulting from heparin injections **(173)** or small hematomas that may mimic cutaneous metastases **(7)** or malignant melanomas **(Fig. 114.2)**. Larger metastases tend to invade the muscles of the abdominal wall **(29)** and often have hypodense, central necrosis **(181)**. Enhancement after intravenous CM may also point to malignancy or a florid inflammatory process. If the degree of CM enhancement is uncertain, a region of interest for densitometric analysis is placed in the lesion on a pre-CM and compared with a post-CM **(Fig. 114.2)**.

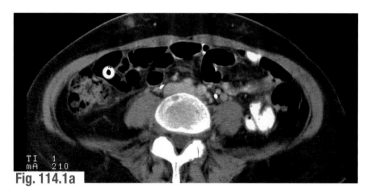

Fig. 114.1a

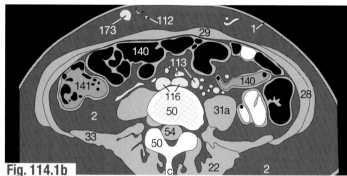

Fig. 114.1b

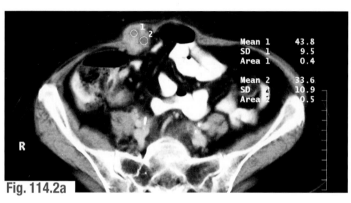

Fig. 114.2a

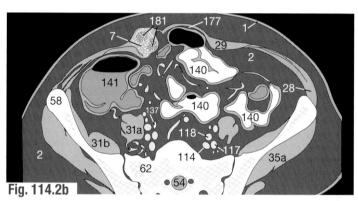

Fig. 114.2b

Metastases in the abdominal wall may not be evident until they become infected and develop into an abscess **(181)** which, in the case illustrated, was catheterized and drained **(182 in Fig. 114.3)**. The second metastasis **(7)**, just beneath the right abdominal wall **(28)**, was not recognized at first because the patient's symptoms were attributed to the adjacent abscess.

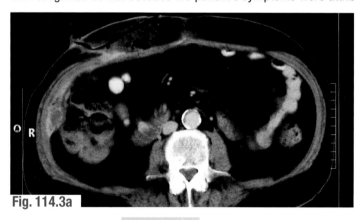

Fig. 114.3a

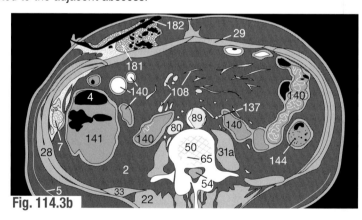

Fig. 114.3b

In elderly patients an inguinal hernia containing small intestine, or even bilateral scrotal hernias containing loops of the small bowel **(140)** may be diagnosed. In the case in **Figure 114.4** the processus vaginalis **(177)** was open bilaterally.

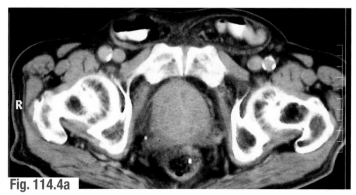

Fig. 114.4a

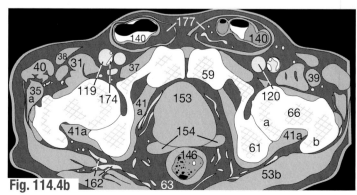

Fig. 114.4b

Segments of the Liver

If a liver biopsy or radiotherapy is planned, it is helpful to know in which segment a focal lesion is situated. The liver is horizontally subdivided (blue line in **Fig. 115.1**) by the main branches of the portal vein **(102)** into a cranial and a caudal part. The main hepatic veins **(103)** mark the borders of the segments in the cranial part **(Fig. 115.2)**. The border between the left and right lobes is <u>not</u> marked by the falciform ligament **(124)**, but by the plane between the middle hepatic vein and gallbladder **(126)** fossa.

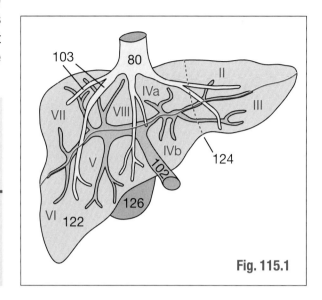

Fig. 115.1

Left lobe	I	caudate lobe
	II	lateral segment, cranial part
	III	lateral segment, caudal part
	IV	quadrate lobe (a: cranial, b: caudal)
Right lobe	V	anterior segment, caudal part
	VI	posterior segment, caudal part
	VII	posterior segment, cranial part
	VIII	anterior segment, cranial part

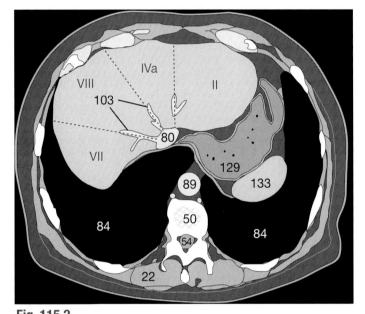

Fig. 115.2

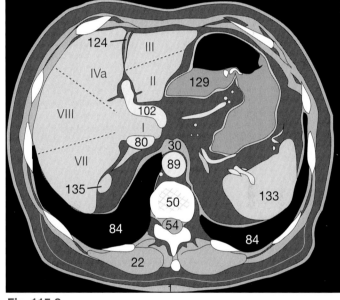

Fig. 115.3

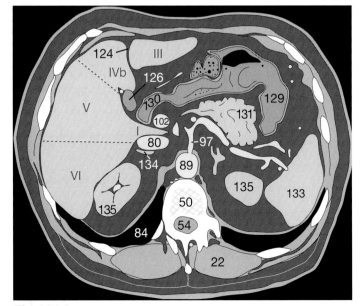

Fig. 115.4

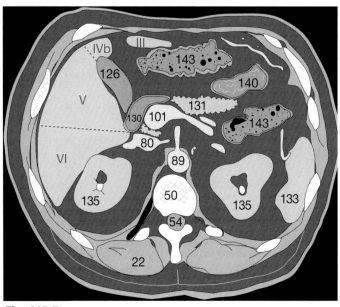

Fig. 115.5

Choice of Window

In conventional (nonhelical) CT the unenhanced liver (122) is imaged on a special liver window width (Fig. 116.1a) set between 120 and 140 HU. Normal liver parenchyma can be more clearly distinguished from lesions on narrow-window-width images because they provide high image contrast. If there is no fatty infiltration of the liver (which would reduce attenuation), intra-hepatic vessels (103) appear as hypodense structures. In cases of fatty infiltration, the veins may appear isodense or even hyper-dense on unenhanced images. The post-CM CT images are viewed using a window width of approximately 350 HU; this smoothes the gray scale contrast (Fig. 116.1c).

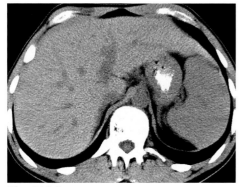

Fig. 116.1a

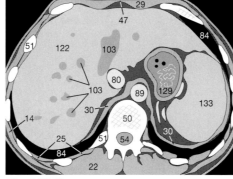

Fig. 116.1b

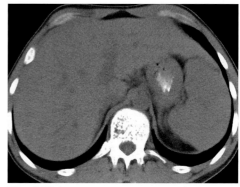

Fig. 116.1c

Passage of a Bolus of Contrast Medium

In a three-phase helical acquisition of early arterial, portal venous, and late venous phases of CM enhancement, an unenhanced study is not necessary [17, 18]. Hypervascular lesions become much more clearly defined in the early arterial phase (Fig. 116.2a) than in the late venous phase. In the late venous (equilibrium) phase (Fig. 116.2b) the density levels of the arterial, portal venous, and venous systems are practically identical.

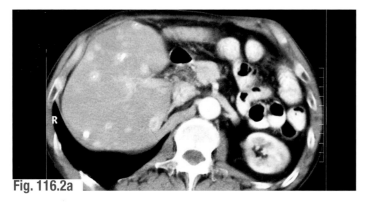

Fig. 116.2a

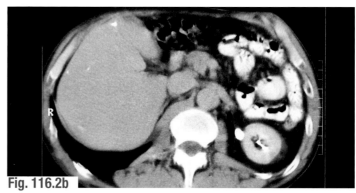

Fig. 116.2b

CT Portography

The chances of demonstrating the true extent of liver lesions (e.g. metastases) are greatly improved if CM is injected directly into the SMA or the splenic artery and images are then acquired in the portal venous phase [17, 21]. Since the principal blood supply for most metastases and tumors comes from the hepatic artery, these lesions will appear hypodense within the hyperdense normal parenchyma that has enhanced with CM (Fig. 116.3a). In the same patient the early arterial phase image (Fig. 116.3b) shows that without CM portography, the extent of the metastases would have been greatly underestimated.

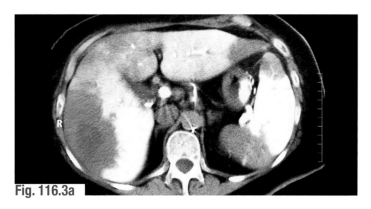

Fig. 116.3a

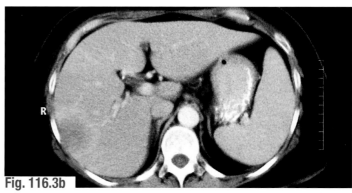

Fig. 116.3b

Hepatic Cysts

Hepatic cysts **(169)** containing serous fluid are sharply defined, thin-walled, homogeneous lesions with density values close to those of water **(Fig. 117.1)**. Partial volume effects may cause poor delineation from adjacent hepatic parenchyma **(122)** if the cysts are small. If in doubt, a ROI should be positioned within the cyst for density measurement **(Fig. 117.2a)**. It is important to ensure the ROI is correctly placed in the center of the cyst, well away from the cyst walls (cf. pp. 11 and 127). In small cysts, for example the poorly defined lesion in **Figure 117.2b**, the average density measurement was too high, because adjacent liver parenchyma was included in the calculation. Note that benign cysts do not show any significant enhancement after i.v. CM.

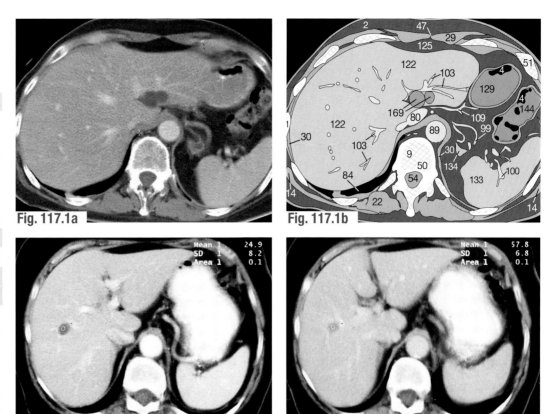

Fig. 117.1a

Fig. 117.1b

Fig. 117.2a

Fig. 117.2b

Hepatic metastases **(7)** may usually be distinguished from benign cysts because they are poorly defined and appear to enhance after i.v. CM (p. 118). In the case illustrated in **Figure 117.3** the mean densities were 55 and 71 HU.

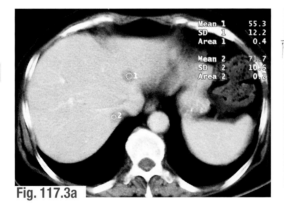

Fig. 117.3a

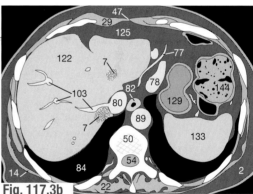

Fig. 117.3b

Hydatid *(Echinococcus granulosus)* cysts have a very characteristic multiloculated appearance, often with radially arranged septations between different cysts (**169** in **Fig. 117.4**). It may prove difficult to differentiate between collapsed, dead cysts and other intrahepatic lesions. The right lobe of the liver is most frequently affected, sometimes the left lobe or the spleen **(133)** become involved, as shown in **Figure 117.4**. The density of the cyst fluid is usually between 10 and 40 HU on an unenhanced image. Partial or complete wall calcification is frequent and the outer membrane may enhance with CM. The DD includes infections with *E. alveolaris* (not shown) and, occasionally, a hepatocellular carcinoma that is poorly defined with irregular satellite lesions.

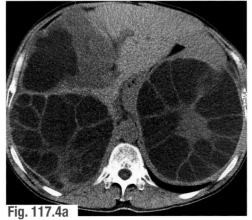

Fig. 117.4a

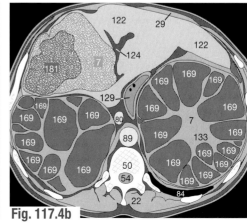

Fig. 117.4b

Liver Metastases

Multiple, focal lesions within the liver suggest metastases. Common sites of origin are the colon, stomach, lung, breast, kidneys, and uterus. The morphology and vascularity differ between the types of liver metastases. An enhanced helical scan is therefore obtained in both the venous phase (**Fig. 118.1a**) and the early arterial phase (**Fig. 118.1c**). In this manner smaller lesions (**7**) become well defined and hepatic veins (**103**) will not be mistaken for metastases.

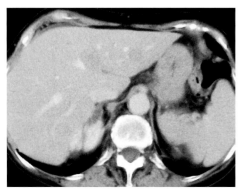

Fig. 118.1a

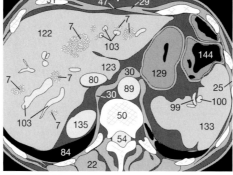

Fig. 118.1b

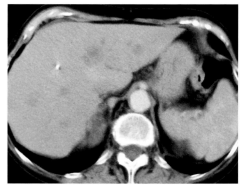

Fig. 118.1c

If helical CT is not available, the diagnosis should be made by comparing an unenhanced scan (**Fig. 118.2**) with an enhanced one (**Fig. 118.3**). In the example shown on the right, the number and size of the lesions (**7**) would have been considerably underestimated if an enhanced scan only had been obtained. The case illustrates the importance of acquiring an unenhanced image. Precontrast images should always be viewed on narrow windows to maximize image contrast within the liver parenchyma (**122**) (cf. p.117). Even small metastases (**7**) might then become visible (**Fig. 118.2**).

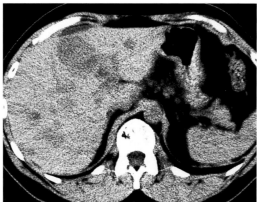

Fig. 118.2a

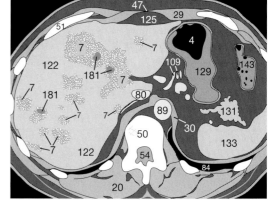

Fig. 118.2b

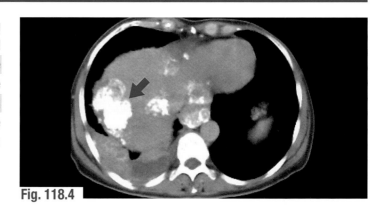

Fig. 118.3a

Fig. 118.3b

In case of diagnostic doubt and for reference at follow-up during therapy, it is useful to compare the CT images with ultrasound findings. Apart from the typical hypoechoic halo, metastases have varied ultrasound appearances, just as in CT images [23]. The ultrasound diagnosis may be difficult especially when calcification in metastases leads to acoustic shadowing. Even though they are quite rare, slowly enlarging mucinous metastases (i.e. those from colon carcinomas) may become very calcified (in **Fig. 118.4**).

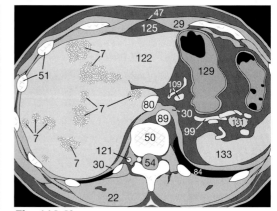

Fig. 118.4

Solid Hepatic Lesions

A hemangioma is the most common benign hepatic lesion. In unenhanced images small hemangioma are well-defined, homogeneous areas of decreased attenuation. After injection of CM, enhancement typically begins in the periphery and progresses toward the center of the hemangioma **(Fig. 119.1a)**, reminiscent of the closing of an optic diaphragm. In dynamic bolus-enhanced CT sequences, enhancement progresses centripetally. Following administration of a CM bolus, a series of CT images is acquired every few seconds at the same location. Accumulation of CM within the cavities of the hemangioma ( ) leads to homogeneous enhancement in the late venous phase **(Fig. 119.1b)**. In large hemangiomas this might take several minutes or be inhomogeneous.

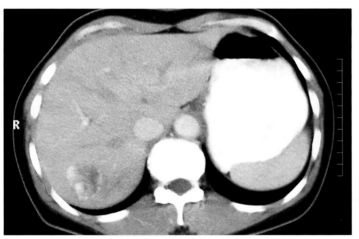

Fig. 119.1a

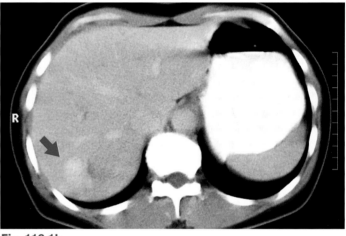

Fig. 119.1b

Hepatic adenoma ( ) occurs most frequently in women between the ages of 20 and 60 who have a long history of taking oral contraceptives. An adenoma originates in hepatocytes and may be solitary or multiple. The adenoma is usually isodense, sometimes hypervascular **(Fig. 119.2)**, and may be accompanied by hypodense infarction, central necrosis, and/or spontaneous, hyperdense hemorrhage. Surgical excision is recommended due to the possibility of acute hemorrhage and malignant degeneration. By contrast, focal nodular hyperplasia (FNH) does not show any tendency of malignant degeneration and lesions of this kind contain biliary ducts. On unenhanced images FNH appears as hypodense, sometimes isodense, but well-defined lesions. After i.v. CM, FNH often demonstrates an irregularly shaped, hypodense, central area (✱) representing its central blood supply; however this feature is seen in only 50% of all FNH **(Fig. 119.3)**.

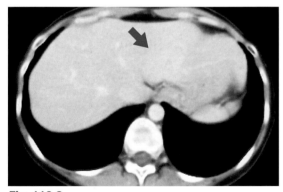

Fig. 119.2

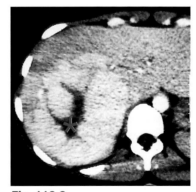

Fig. 119.3

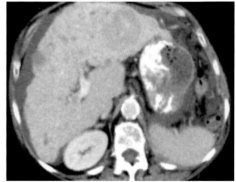

Fig. 119.4

Hepatocellular carcinoma (HCC) often occurs in patients who have a long history of hepatic cirrhosis and is seen most often in men over the age of 40. In one-third of all cases HCC is solitary although multifocal lesions are not rare. Thromboses in the branches of the portal vein caused by tumor invasion into the lumen of the vessel may be seen in one-third of cases. The CT appearance of HCC **(Fig. 119.4)** is extremely variable. On unenhanced images HCC usually appears hypodense or isodense; CM may show diffuse or rim enhancement and central necrosis. When there is also cirrhosis, it may be difficult to define the border of an HCC.

Secondary lymphoma should be considered in the DD because it may infiltrate the liver parenchyma and may be the cause of diffuse hepatomegaly. Of course this does not mean that every case of hepatomegaly is due to a lymphoma. NonHodgkin's lymphomas resemble HCC because of their similarities in vascularity and nodular growth.

Diffuse Hepatic Lesions

In fatty changes of the liver, the density of the unenhanced parenchyma, which is normally about 65 HU, may reduce so that it is either isodense, or even hypodense with regard to the blood vessels (**Fig. 120.1**; cf. also p. 116). In hemochromatosis (**Fig. 120.2**) the accumulation of iron leads to increased attenuation above 90 HU and may reach as much as 140 HU. In these cases the natural contrast between parenchyma and vessels is even greater. Cirrhosis (**Fig. 120.3**), resulting from chronic liver damage, has a diffuse nodular appearance and usually gives the organ an irregular, lumpy contour.

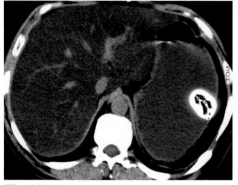
Fig. 120.1

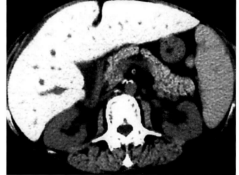
Fig. 120.2

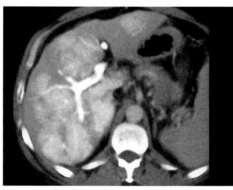
Fig. 120.3

Abdominal Pathology — Gallbladder

Biliary Tract

After surgical choledochoenteric anastomosis, sphincterotomy, or endoscopic retrograde cholangiopancreatography (ERCP), hypodense gas (➡) is usually present within the intrahepatic bile ducts (**Fig. 120.4**). These causes of biliary gas must be differentiated from gas-forming anaerobic bacteria within an abscess.
Dilatation of the intrahepatic biliary tract (**128**) is called cholestasis (**Fig. 120.5**). It may result from gallstones, a malignant obstruc-

tion of the biliary tract or from a pancreatic carcinoma at Vater's ampulla. In **Figure 120.5**, note the calcification (**174**) of the tortuous splenic artery (**99**) and the hepatic metastases (**7**). These poorly defined and only slightly hypodense metastases must be differentiated from artifacts (**3**) arising from the ribs adjacent to the liver (**122**) and spleen (**133**). These beam-hardening artifacts result from the abrupt changes in attenuation between the viscera and the rib (**51**).

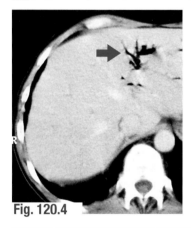
Fig. 120.4

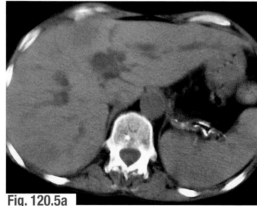
Fig. 120.5a

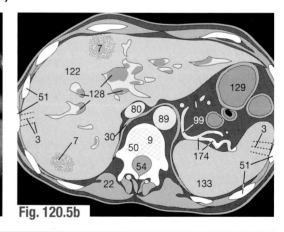
Fig. 120.5b

If it is not possible to treat the cause of cholestasis surgically, inserting a stent (**182** in **Fig. 120.6**) may decompress an obstructed biliary duct (**128**).

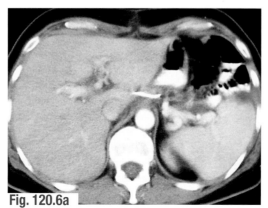
Fig. 120.6a

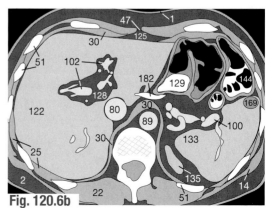
Fig. 120.6b

The size and shape of the gallbladder vary depending on when the patient last ate food. A hydrops of the gallbladder should only be diagnosed if there is very marked dilatation, that is if the diameter exceeds 5 cm in several transverse planes. The attenuation of bile is usually just greater than that of water (0 HU) but may increase to up to 25 HU if the bile is highly concentrated [4].

Cholecystolithiasis

Stones **(167)** within the gallbladder **(126)** may show different patterns of calcification **(Fig. 121.1)**. Cup-shaped and ring-like calcifications can be seen in stones containing cholesterol and bilirubin **(Fig. 121.2)**. If stones obstruct gallbladder drainage or inflammation has caused a stenosis, sludge may form resulting in increased attenuation and sedimentation of bile **(Fig. 121.3)**. Common duct stones can be diagnosed using thin-section CT because smaller stones might be missed in standard thickness sections.

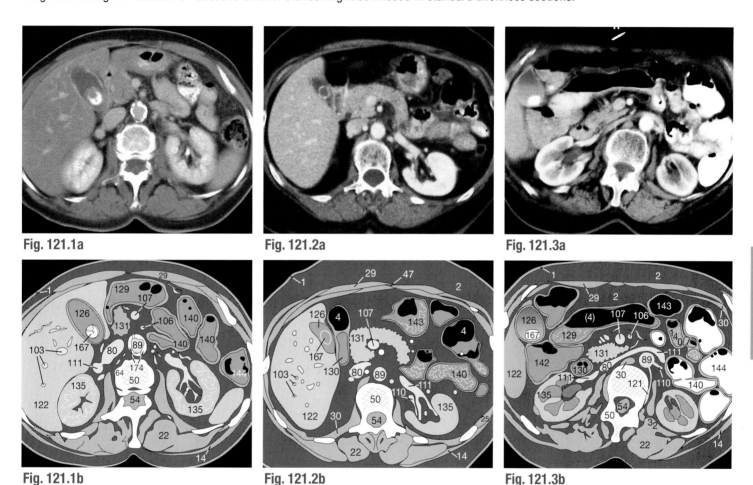

Fig. 121.1a   Fig. 121.2a   Fig. 121.3a

Fig. 121.1b   Fig. 121.2b   Fig. 121.3b

Chronic Inflammatory Lesions

Cholecystolithiasis can lead to chronic inflammation, resulting in either a stone-filled, shrunken gallbladder, or acute cholecystitis or an empyema of the gallbladder (recognized by an irregularly thickened wall) (↖ ↗ in **Fig. 121.4**). There is an increased risk of malignant change with chronic inflammatory processes [24]. The development of a porcelain gallbladder **(Fig. 121.5)** with an egg-shell-like pattern of calcification **(174)** may be a premalignant lesion.

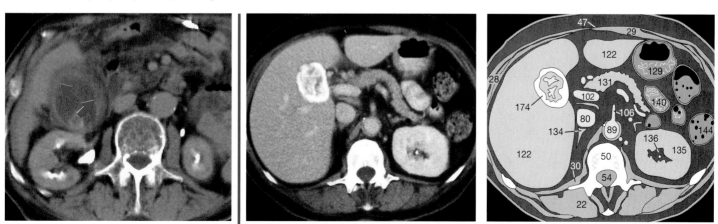

Fig. 121.4   Fig. 121.5a   Fig. 121.5b

Contrast Enhancement

Before reading further, try to define a characteristic feature of the spleen by looking at **Figure 122.1a**. The normal splenic parenchyma **(133)** has an attenuation of approximately 45 HU on unenhanced images. The attenuation of the spleen will only appear homogeneous in an unenhanced image or in the late venous phase of an enhanced study **(Fig. 122.1c)**. In the early arterial phase **(Fig. 122.1a)** it will enhance heterogeneously and appear patchy or marbled, a pattern representing its trabecular architecture. This pattern should not be misinterpreted as an abnormality. Note also the uneven distribution of CM within the inferior vena cava **(80)** and the two (!) hepatic metastases **(7)** in the same image **(Fig. 122.1a)**. Did you spot the areas of near-water attenuation representing perisplenic/perihepatic ascites **(8)**?

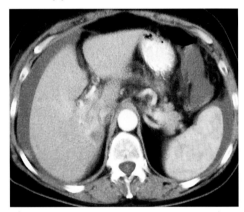

Fig. 122.1a

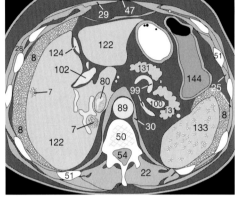

Fig. 122.1b

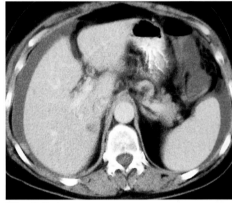

Fig. 122.1c

The splenic artery **(99)** is typically elongated and tortuous so that it may be imaged in several consecutive slices. In elderly patients it is common to see atherosclerotic plaques **(174** in **Fig. 122.2)**. Occasionally a homogeneous splenunculus [accessory spleen ↗], well demonstrated in the surrounding fat, may be seen at the hilum or the inferior pole of the spleen **(Fig. 122.3)**. Differentiating between a splenunculus and an abnormally enlarged LN may be difficult.

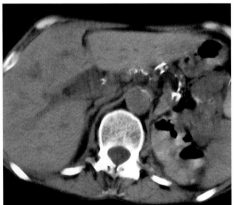

Fig. 122.2a

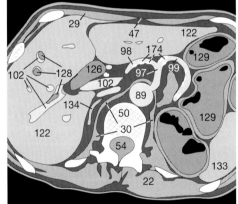

Fig. 122.2b

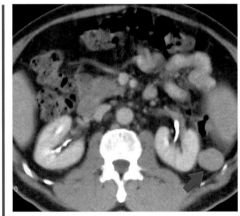

Fig. 122.3

Splenomegaly

Diffuse enlargement of the spleen **(Fig. 123.1)** may be caused by several conditions: portal hypertension, leukemia/lymphoma, myelofibrosis and hemolytic anemia, or by various storage diseases. Assessment of splenic size is made difficult by individual variations in shape. Marked splenomegaly is easily recognized, but in borderline cases of splenomegaly and for follow-up one should know the normal range of splenic size. In the transverse plane the length of the spleen should measure no more than 10 cm (dotted line) and its width (**d**, at right angles to the dotted line) should not exceed 5 cm **(Fig. 122.4)**.

In ultrasound, the spleen is not measured in a transverse plane but in an oblique plane parallel to the intercostal space. In this plane the upper limit of normal is 11 cm for the long axis [28].

The craniocaudal dimension of the spleen should not exceed 15 cm, so that at a slice thickness of 1 cm it should not be visible on more than 15 sections. Splenomegaly is diagnosed if at least two of these three parameters are exceeded.

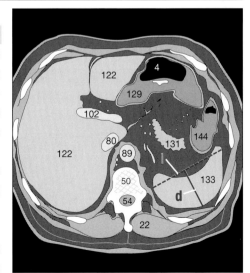

Fig. 122.4

As splenomegaly develops, the typical normal crescentic shape is lost **(Fig. 123.1)**. Gross splenomegaly, which may be caused by chronic lymphocytic leukemia, acts as a space-occupying mass and displaces adjacent organs. In **Figure 123.1** the left kidney is compressed (⬇). If the blood supply cannot keep pace with splenic growth, infarctions (↙) may result. These appear as hypodense areas that do not enhance with CM **(Fig. 123.2)**.

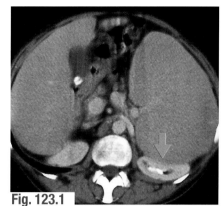

Fig. 123.1

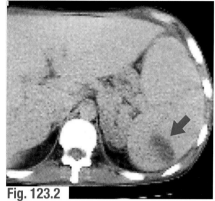

Fig. 123.2

Focal Splenic Lesions

Splenic cysts share the same characteristics of hepatic cysts (cf. p.117). Metastases in the spleen **(7)** are rare and difficult to distinguish from cysts. In the case illustrated in **Figure 123.3**, the diagnosis of splenic metastases was relatively easy because there were hepatic lesions and malignant ascites **(8)**. If there are multifocal lesions with inhomogeneous CM enhancement, a diagnosis of focal splenic lymphoma or splenic candidiasis should be considered. Ascites **(8)** may accompany candidiasis, as shown in **Figure 123.4**. Splenic lymphoma is usually characterized by diffuse infiltration and the spleen may appear normal.

The examination of the spleen **(133)** after a blunt thoracic or abdominal trauma must be meticulous. Lacerations of the parenchyma **(181)** may lead to hematomas **(8)** beneath the capsule, and delayed rupture of the capsule may cause massive hemorrhage into the abdominal cavity **(Fig. 123.5)**.

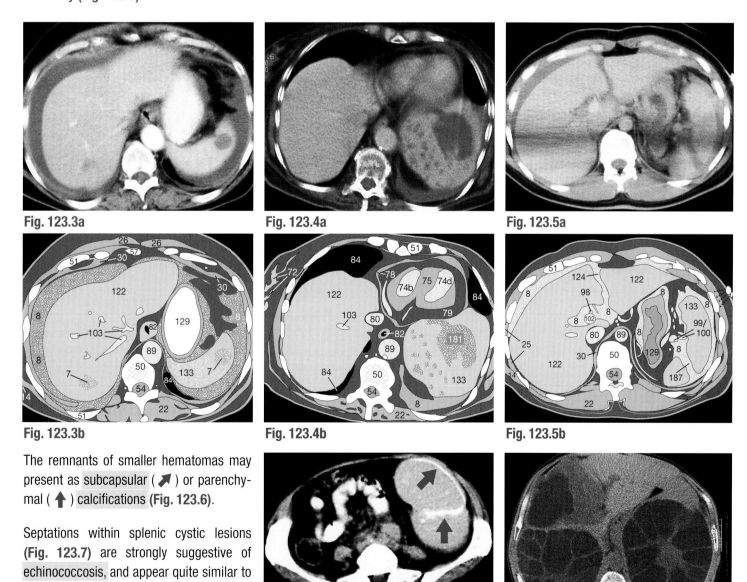

Fig. 123.3a **Fig. 123.4a** **Fig. 123.5a**

Fig. 123.3b **Fig. 123.4b** **Fig. 123.5b**

The remnants of smaller hematomas may present as subcapsular (↗) or parenchymal (⬆) calcifications **(Fig. 123.6)**.

Septations within splenic cystic lesions **(Fig. 123.7)** are strongly suggestive of echinococcosis, and appear quite similar to those in the liver. In most cases the liver is also affected (cf. p.117).

Fig. 123.6 **Fig. 123.7**

Acute and Chronic Pancreatitis

Acute pancreatitis may present as edematous interstitial pancreatitis (**Fig. 124.1**). Hypodense peripancreatic fluid (exudate) **(8)** and edema of the connective tissue **(185)** are frequent findings. CT shows blurring of the pancreatic contours; the normally lobular pattern of the pancreas is effaced (**Figs. 124.1** and **124.2**). In hemorrhagic necrotizing pancreatitis (**Fig. 124.2**) the extent of necrosis is a prognostic feature.

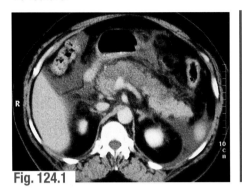
Fig. 124.1

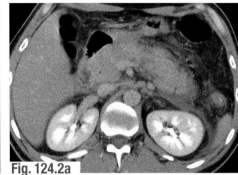
Fig. 124.2a

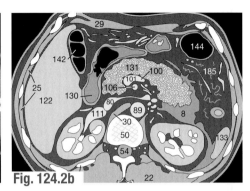
Fig. 124.2b

Chronic pancreatitis progresses either slowly and progressively or in recurrent episodes. The two most common causes of chronic pancreatitis are alcohol abuse and cholelithiasis.

Typical findings in chronic pancreatitis are fibrosis and multifocal calcifications **(174)**, irregular dilatation of the pancreatic duct **(132)**, and sometimes the formation of pseudocysts **(169)** within, or next to, the pancreas **(131)** (**Figs. 124.3** and **124.4**). The disease may lead to pancreatic atrophy as a late feature. The possibility that pancreatic carcinoma develops in association with chronic, calcific pancreatitis is presently being discussed.

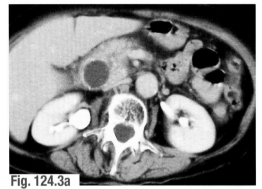
Fig. 124.3a

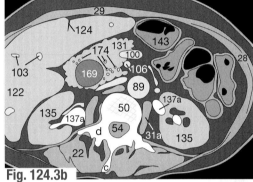
Fig. 124.3b

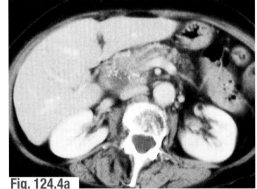
Fig. 124.4a

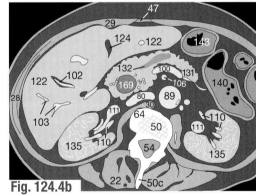
Fig. 124.4b

Pancreatic Neoplasms

Most pancreatic carcinomas **(7)** are located within the head of the pancreas **(131)**. As a result, even small tumors may cause cholestasis by obstructing the common bile duct **(127)** (**Fig. 124.5**). Pancreatic carcinomas tend to metastasize very early to the liver and the regional LNs. In case of doubt, ERCP should be carried out to image the pancreatic and common bile ducts. Islet cell tumors, 75% of which are functional, are located within the body of the pancreas. The Zollinger-Ellison syndrome (**Fig. 124.6**) is caused by a gastrin-secreting tumor (✎). Other neoplasms associated with the pancreas are insulinomas, glucagonomas, and serotonin-producing masses.

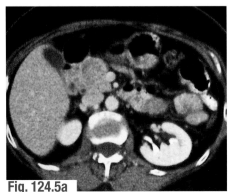
Fig. 124.5a

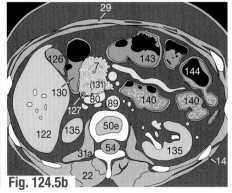
Fig. 124.5b

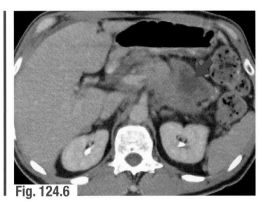
Fig. 124.6

The normal position and shape of the adrenal glands has been described on pages 83 to 84. The maximum lengths of the adrenal glands range between 2.1 and 2.7 cm, the right adrenal often being somewhat longer than the left. The thickness of the limbs should not exceed 5 to 8 mm in the transverse plane. A fusiform or nodular thickening **(7)** is likely to be abnormal in CT, and is usually indicative of hyperplasia or an adenoma of the adrenal gland (**134** in **Fig. 125.1**). Typically, the adrenals can be clearly differentiated from adjacent fat, the diaphragm **(30)**, the kidney **(135)**, the liver **(122)**, and the inferior vena cava **(80)**.

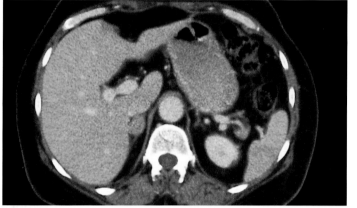

Fig. 125.1a

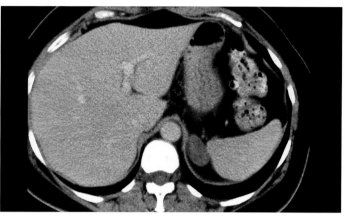

Fig. 125.2a

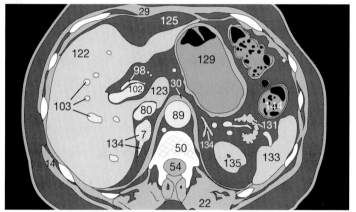

Fig. 125.1b

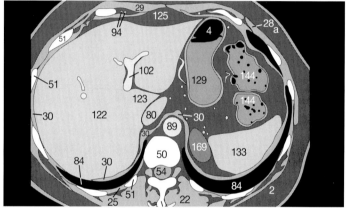

Fig. 125.2b

The following conditions may be dignosed according to the specific hormonal excess; congenital adrenal cortical hyperplasia (androgens), Conn's syndrome (aldosterone) and Cushing's syndrome (cortisone). An upper pole renal cyst or a renal angiomyolipoma (cf. **Fig. 128.4**) must be included in the DD. Attenuation values for benign cysts **(169)** should lie close to those for water (= −1 HU in the present case) **(Fig. 125.2)**. (Compare with cysts on p. 127.)

In cases of heterogeneous enlargement of the adrenal gland or infiltration of adjacent organs, a metastasis or a carcinoma (**Fig. 125.3**) must be suspected. Since bronchogenic carcinomas often metastasize to the liver and the adrenals, staging chest CT studies for lung cancer should be extended to include the caudal margin of the liver and the adrenals. Tumors of the paravertebral sympathetic trunks, which are located close to the adrenal glands, may also be detected, but they are rare. The MRI images in **Figures 125.4a** and **125.4b** show a neuroblastoma (➡) in the sagittal (a) and coronal (b) planes.

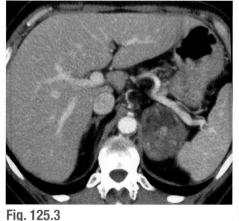

Fig. 125.3

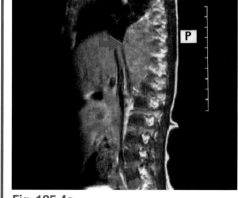

Fig. 125.4a

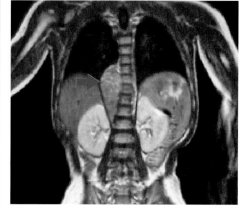

Fig. 125.4b

Congenital Variations

The attenuation of the renal parenchyma **(135)** on unenhanced images is approximately 30 HU. The kidneys occasionally develop to different sizes. If the outlines are smooth and the parenchymal thickness is not irregular, it is likely to represent unilateral renal hypoplasia **(Fig. 126.1)**. The smaller kidney need not be abnormal.

A kidney may have an atypical orientation as in **Figure 126.2**. However, if a kidney lies in the iliac fossa **(Fig. 126.3)**, this does not indicate an ectopic location, but a renal transplant **(135)**. The organ is connected to the iliac vessels **(113/116)** and the urinary bladder **(138)**.

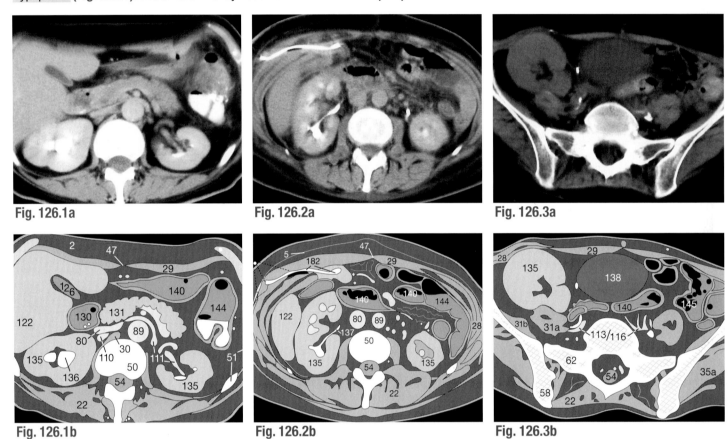

Fig. 126.1a

Fig. 126.2a

Fig. 126.3a

Fig. 126.1b

Fig. 126.2b

Fig. 126.3b

Marked differences in size, as in **Figure 126.2**, may indicate partial or complete renal duplication on one side. The positions and number of renal arteries may vary considerably (**110** in **Fig. 126.1b**). The renal arteries must be examined carefully for evidence of stenosis as a cause of renal hypertension. The ureter (137 ➡) can be present as a partial or complete duplex ureter. In complete renal duplication, the renal pelvis is also duplicated.

Occasionally the low-density fat in the hilum (✱ in **Fig. 126.5b**) is only poorly demarcated from the renal parenchyma **(135)** owing to a beam-hardening artifact or partial volume averaging **(Fig. 126.5a)**. This gives the incorrect impression of a renal tumor. Comparison with an immediately adjacent section **(Fig. 126.5c)** demonstrates that only hilar fat was present. The actual tumor in this particular example **(7)** is situated at the posterior margin of the right lobe of the liver **(122)**.

Fig. 126.4

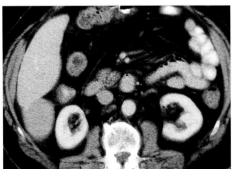

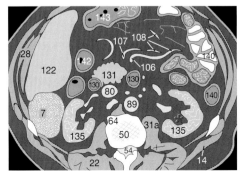

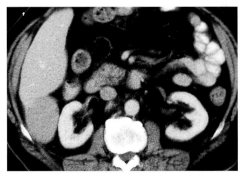

Fig. 126.5a

Fig. 126.5b

Fig. 126.5c

Cysts

Renal cysts are frequent incidental findings in adults and may be located anywhere in the parenchyma. They may be exophytic or parapelvic, in which case they can resemble a hydronephrosis. Benign cysts contain a serous, usually clear liquid with an attenuation of between −5 and +15 HU. They do not enhance with CM because they are avascular. The attenuation measurement may be inaccurate if there are partial volume averaging artifacts due to slice thickness (**Fig. 127.1**: ca. 25 HU) or to eccentric positioning of the ROI (**Fig. 127.2**: ca. 22 HU) (cf. pp. 11 and 12). Only the correct positioning of the ROI in the center of the cyst (○ in **Fig. 127.3**) will provide an accurate average of 10 HU. In rare cases hemorrhage into benign cysts will result in hyperdense values on unenhanced images. The attenuation values will not change on post-contrast images.

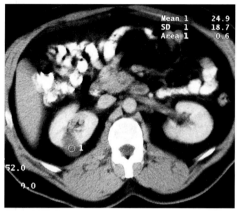 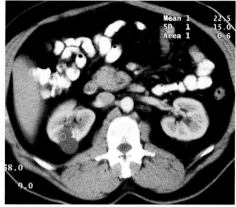 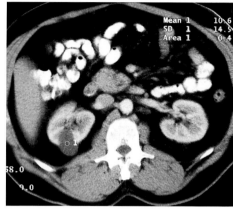

Fig. 127.1   Fig. 127.2   Fig. 127.3

Increased density or calcifications in a mass may indicate past renal tuberculosis, current Echinococcus infestation (hydatid disease), or a cystic renal cell carcinoma. The difference between pre- and post-contrast images also provides information on renal function: after approximately 30 seconds the well-perfused renal cortex is the first part of the kidney to accumulate the CM (cf. **Figs. 127.2** and **127.3**). After another 30 to 60 seconds the CM is excreted into the more distal tubules leading to enhancement of the medulla. The result is homogeneous enhancement of the renal parenchyma (cf. **Fig. 127.1**).

The appearances of multiple renal cysts in children with congenital autosomal recessive polycystic kidney disease are dramatically different from those of the occasional cysts found in adults, which are generally incidental findings. Polycystic kidney disease in the adult (**169** in **Fig. 127.4**) is autosomal dominant and associated with multiple cysts of the liver, the bile ducts and, more rarely, with cysts in the pancreas or with abdominal or cerebral aneurysms.

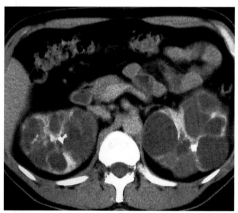 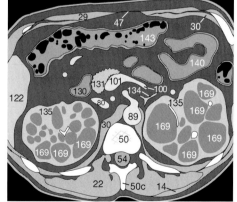 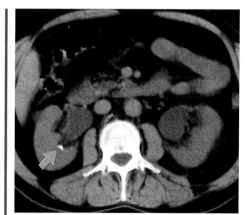

Fig. 127.4a   Fig. 127.4b   Fig. 127.5

Hydronephrosis

Parapelvic cysts may be confused with grade 1 hydronephrosis (**Fig. 127.5**), which is characterized in the unenhanced image by a dilated renal pelvis and ureter. In grade 2 hydronephrosis the renal calyces become poorly defined. When parenchymal atrophy ensues, the hydronephrosis is categorized as grade 3 (see p. 128). Since no CM had been given to the patient in **Figure 127.5**, the hyperdense lesion (↗) in the right kidney must be a renal calculus.

For the diagnosis of nephrolithiasis alone, CT should be avoided because of undue radiation exposure. Sonography is the method of choice for nephrolithiasis as well as hydronephrosis.

Hydronephrosis, which causes dilatation of the ureter **(137)** and the renal pelvis **(136)**, impairs renal function **(Fig. 128.1)**. In this image the left renal parenchyma **(135)** shows delayed and reduced CM enhancement as compared with the normal, right kidney.

Chronic, grade 3 hydronephrosis reduces the parenchyma to a narrow rim of tissue **(Fig. 128.2)**, resulting finally in atrophy and a non-functioning kidney. In cases of doubt, identifying the dilated ureter (↘ in **Fig. 128.2b**) can resolve the DD between a parapelvic cyst and hydronephrosis. CM accumulates in a dilated renal pelvis, but not in a cyst.

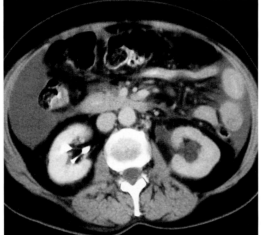

Fig. 128.1a

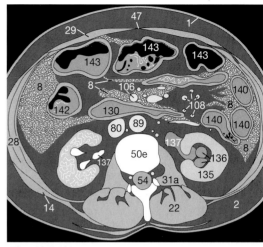

Fig. 128.1b

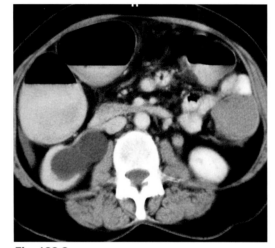

Fig. 128.2a

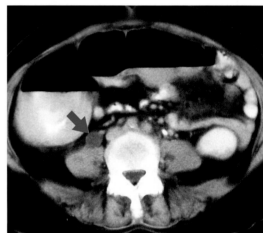

Fig. 128.2b

Solid Tumors

Enhancement with CM often helps to distinguish between partial volume averaging of benign renal cysts and hypodense renal tumors, since CT morphology alone does not provide sufficient information about the etiology of a lesion. This is especially so when a mass (✱) is poorly defined within the parenchyma **(Fig. 128.3)**. Inhomogeneous enhancement, infiltration of adjacent structures, and invasion of the pelvis or the renal vein are criteria of malignancy.

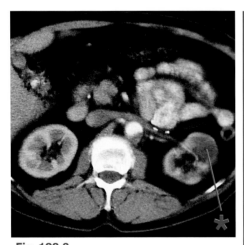

Fig. 128.3

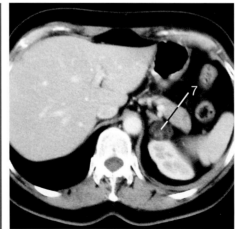

Fig. 128.4

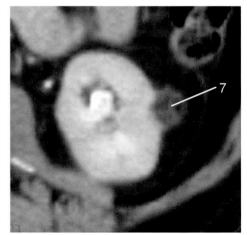

Fig. 128.5

However, when a mass consists not only of solid, inhomogeneous areas, but also contains fat, an angiomyolipoma **(7)** must be considered **(Figs. 128.4 and 128.5)**. These benign hamartomas contain fat, atypical muscle fibers and blood vessels. The vessel walls are abnormal, and the complication of intratumoral or retroperitoneal hemorrhage may occur (not depicted here).

Kidney Problems Related to Blood Vessels

If ultrasound shows fresh hemorrhage into the abdomen after penetration or blunt trauma, the source of bleeding must be located as soon as possible. The DD must include not only splenic rupture or major vessel disruption but also renal injury. On unenhanced images of a renal rupture (**Figs. 129.1a** and **129.1b**) the contours of the kidney (**135**) appear blurred and, depending on the extent of hemorrhage, hyperdense fresh hematoma (**8**) can be detected in the retroperitoneal spaces. In this case enhanced images (**Figs. 129.1c** and **129.1b**) show that the renal parenchyma (**135**) is still well perfused and function is maintained.

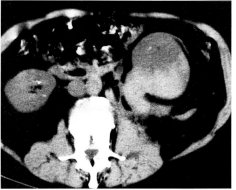
Fig. 129.1a

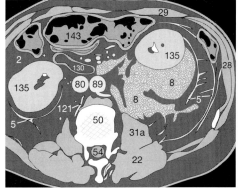
Fig. 129.1b

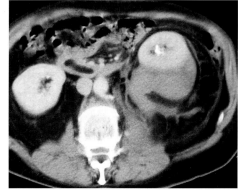
Fig. 129.1c

After extracorporeal shock-wave lithotripsy (ESWL), renal injuries may rarely occur that lead to small hematomas or extravasation of urine from the ureter. If there is hematuria or persisting pain after ESWL, it is essential to obtain delayed images. Urine leaking into the retroperitoneal spaces (➡ in **Figs. 129.2a** through **129.2c**) would not be opacified in images obtained before the kidney has excreted CM.

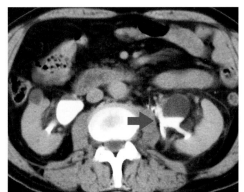
Fig. 129.2a

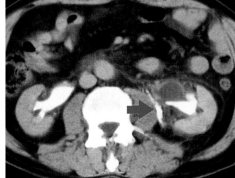
Fig. 129.2b

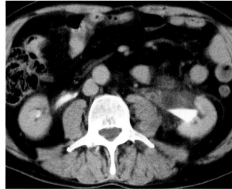
Fig. 129.2c

Renal infarctions (**180**) usually have a triangular shape on CT images corresponding to the vascular architecture of the kidney (**Fig. 129.3**). The broad base abuts the capsule and the triangle gradually tapers toward the pelvis (**136**). A typical feature is the lack of enhancement after i.v. CM in the early perfusion phase and in the late excretion phase. Embolisms usually originate in the left heart, or in the aorta in cases of atherosclerosis (**174** in **Fig. 129.3**) or aneurysms (cf. p. 136).

If there is a low attenuation filling defect (**173**) in the lumen of the renal vein (**111**) after a CM injection, the presence of bland thrombus (**Fig. 129.4**) or tumor thrombus from a renal carcinoma extending into the inferior vena cava (**80**) must be considered.

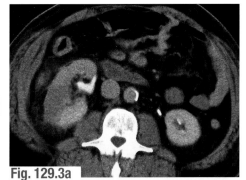
Fig. 129.3a

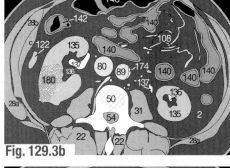
Fig. 129.3b

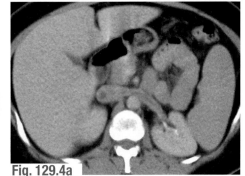
Fig. 129.4a

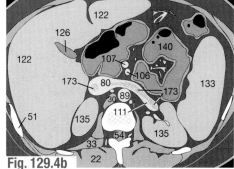
Fig. 129.4b

Catheters

The walls of the urinary bladder are best examined if the bladder is distended. If a urinary catheter (182) is in place at the time of CT (Fig. 130.1), sterile water can be instilled as a low-density CM. Focal or diffuse wall thickening of a trabeculated bladder, associated with prostatic hyperplasia, will be demonstrated clearly. If a ureter (137) has been stented (182) for strictures or retroperitoneal tumors, the distal end of the JJ stent (138) may be visible in the bladder lumen (bilateral JJ stents in Fig. 130.2).

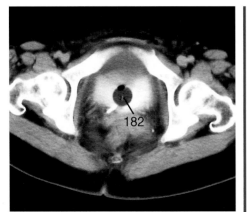

Fig. 130.1

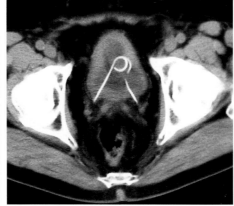

Fig. 130.2a

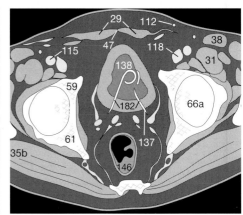

Fig. 130.2b

Diverticula

Diverticula situated at the periphery of the bladder can easily be distinguished from ovarian cysts by using CM (Fig. 130.3). The "jet phenomenon" is often seen in the posterior basal recess of the bladder and is caused by peristalsis in the ureters. They inject spurts of CM-opacified urine into the bladder, which is filled with hypodense urine (Fig. 130.4).

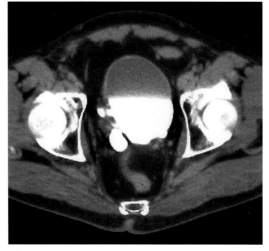

Fig. 130.3

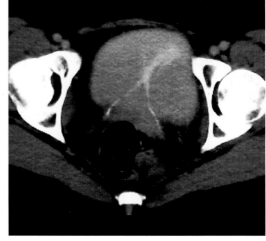

Fig. 130.4

Solid Tumors

Bladder wall tumors (7), which become visible after intravenous or intravesical CM, have characteristic, irregular margins that do not enhance with CM (Fig. 130.5). Tumors must not be confused with intravesicular blood clots that may occur following transurethral resection of the prostate. It is important to determine the precise size of the tumor and to what extent adjacent organs (e.g., cervix, uterus, or rectum) have been infiltrated (◀ in Fig. 130.6).

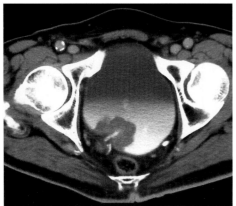

Fig. 130.5a

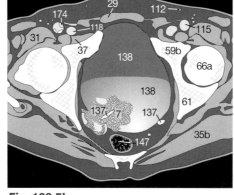

Fig. 130.5b

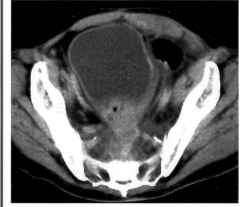

Fig. 130.6

If the bladder has been resected because of carcinoma, a urinary reservoir (★) can be constructed using a loop of small bowel (ileum conduit) which has been isolated from the GIT. Urine is excreted from the reservoir into a urostomy bag (⬅ in **Fig. 131.1b**). In **Figure 131.2** a colostomy (⬇) is also seen (cf. p. 134).

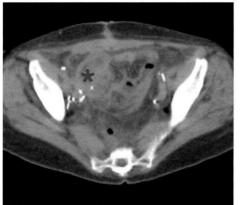

Fig. 131.1a

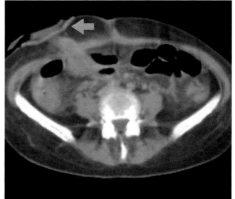

Fig. 131.1b

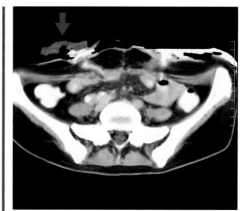

Fig. 131.2

Abdominal Pathology

Reproductive Organs

Uterus

Foreign bodies in the uterine cavity **(158)**, e.g. an intrauterine contraceptive device **(166)**, are not always as clearly visible in a transverse image as in **Figure 131.3**. Calcifications **(174)** are a characteristic feature of benign uterine myomas. Nevertheless it can be difficult to distinguish multiple myomas from a carcinoma of the uterus (**7** in **Fig. 131.4**). If the adjacent walls of the bladder **(138)** or the rectum **(146)** are infiltrated, the tumor is most likely to be malignant **(Fig. 131.5)**. Central necrosis **(181)** occurs in both kinds of tumors and is usually indicative of a rapidly growing, that is malignant tumor **(Fig. 131.4)**.

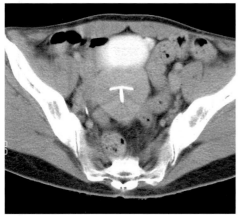

Fig. 131.3a

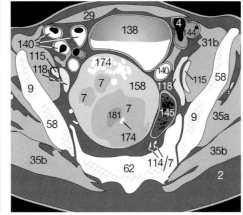

Fig. 131.4a

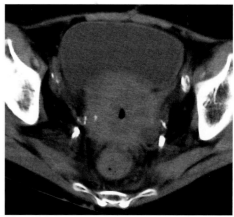

Fig. 131.5a

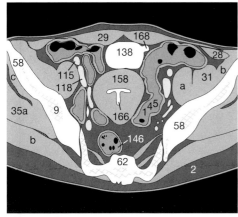

Fig. 131.3b

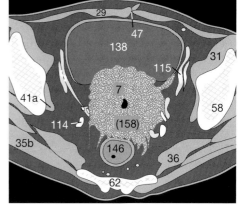

Fig. 131.4b

Fig. 131.5b

Ovaries

The most common ovarian lesions are thin-walled follicular cysts **(169)** which contain a clear fluid with a density equivalent to that of water, that is below 15 HU **(Fig. 132.1)**. Density measurements, however, are unreliable in small cysts (cf. p. 127). These cannot be clearly differentiated from mucinous cysts or hemorrhagic cysts. This latter type of cyst may be caused by endometriosis. Sometimes cysts reach considerable sizes **(Fig. 132.2)** with consequent mass effect.

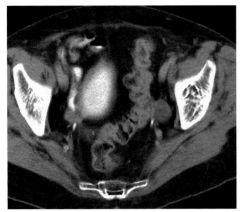

Fig. 132.1a

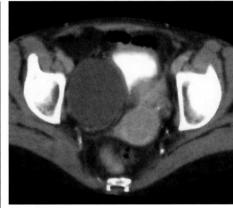

Fig. 132.1b

Fig. 132.2

The malignant nature of solid ovarian tumors can be suspected if there are the following general criteria used for other tumors:
1) ill-defined margins;
2) infiltration of adjacent structures;
3) enlarged regional LNs; and
4) inhomogeneous enhancement with CM.
Peritoneal carcinomatosis **(Fig. 132.3)** frequently occurs in advanced ovarian carcinoma, and is characterized by the appearance of multiple fine nodules and edema **(185)** in the greater omentum, the root of the mesenteric, the abdominal wall, and by ascites **(8)**.

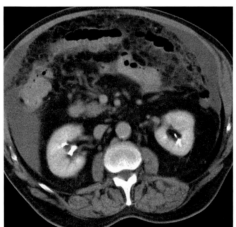

Fig. 132.3a

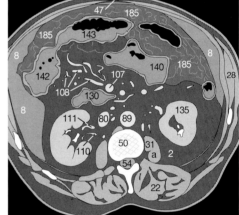

Fig. 132.3b

Prostate, Vas Deferens

High-density calcification representing postinflammatory residue is often encountered following prostatitis **(Fig. 132.4)**. Calcifications are also occasionally seen in the vas deferens **(Fig. 132.5)**. Carcinoma of the prostate is only detectable in advanced stages **(Fig. 132.6)** when the bladder wall or the adjacent ischiorectal fossa fat are infiltrated. If a prostate carcinoma is suspected, all images should be carefully viewed on bone windows for sclerotic metastases (see p. 139).

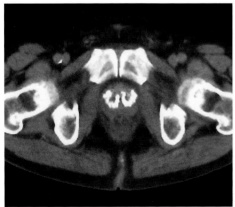

Fig. 132.4

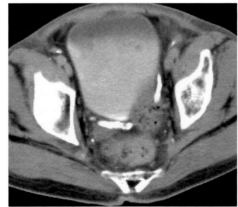

Fig. 132.5

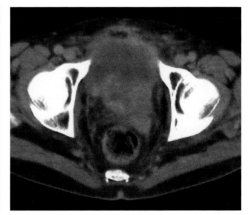

Fig. 132.6

Stomach

Despite the advantages of using water as a hypodense CM for imaging the stomach after intravenous Buscopan [15, 16], small tumors may escape detection during conventional CTs. Endoscopy and endosonography should be employed to complement CT. Marked focal wall thickening, which occurs in carcinoma of the stomach, is usually easily recognized (⬅ in Fig. 133.1). In cases of diffuse wall thickening, the DD should also include lymphoma, leiomyoma, or leiomyosarkoma of the stomach. It is vital to look for bubbles of intraperitoneal gas, which is evidence of a small perforation (↙ in Fig. 133.3) possibly occuring with ulcers or advanced ulcerating carcinomas.

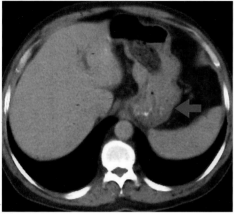

Fig. 133.1

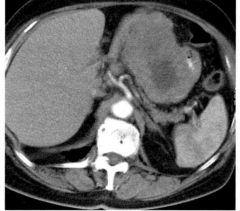

Fig. 133.2

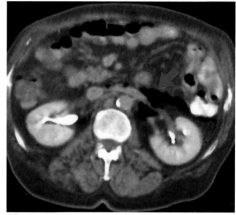

Fig. 133.3

Inflammation of the Intestines

The entire small and large bowel must be examined for wall thickening or infiltration of the surrounding fat, as per the checklist on page 81. Both ulcerative colitis (Fig. 133.4) and Crohn's disease (Fig. 133.5) are characterized by thickening of the affected bowel wall (↑) so that several layers of the wall may become visible. Disseminated intravascular coagulopathy (DIC) or over-anticoagulation with warfarin may cause diffuse hemorrhage (8) in the bowel wall (140) and also lead to mural thickening (Fig. 133.6). The DD should include ischemia if the abnormality is limited to segments in the territory of the mesenteric vessels, for example in the walls of the colon (152), as a result of advanced atherosclerosis (174) or an embolus (Fig. 133.7). You should therefore check that the mesenteric vessels (108) and the walls of the intestine enhance homogeneously after i.v. CM.

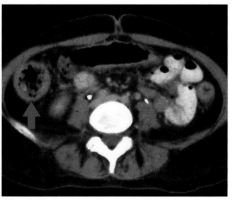

Fig. 133.4

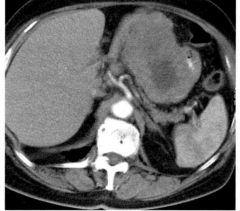

Fig. 133.6a

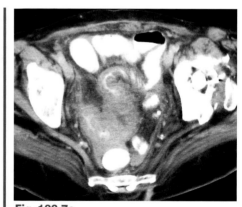

Fig. 133.7a

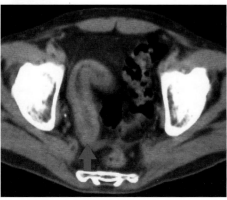

Fig. 133.5

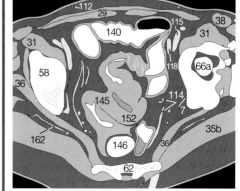

Fig. 133.6b

Fig. 133.7b

Colon

Elderly patients frequently have diverticular disease **(168)** of the descending colon **(144)** and sigmoid colon (**145** in **Fig. 134.1**). The condition is more significant if acute diverticulitis has developed **(Fig. 134.2)**, which is characterized by ill-defined colonic walls and by edematous infiltration of the surrounding mesenteric fat (↘ in **Fig. 134.2**).

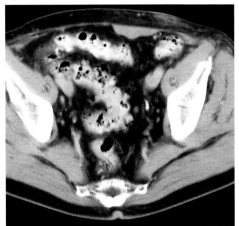

Fig. 134.1a

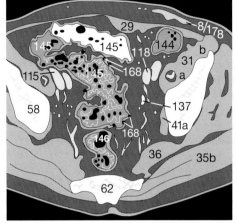

Fig. 134.1b

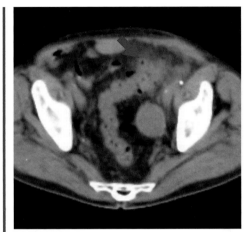

Fig. 134.2

Malignant thickening of the colonic wall (**152** in **Fig. 134.3**) is not always easily distinguished from that found in colitis (cf. p. 133): in both conditions there is stranding of the pericolic fat. The liver should always be checked for metastases if the cause of the colonic abnormality is uncertain.

A temporary colostomy (**170** in **Fig. 134.4**) may be necessary if a left hemicolectomy or sigmoid colectomy was performed because of perforated diverticulitis or carcinoma. The colostomy is permanent if the rectum was excised. A potential complication of a colostomy can be seen in **Figure 134.5**: there is an abscess in the abdominal wall **(181)**. A carcinoid lesion of the small bowel (↙ in **Fig. 134.6**) may simulate a carcinoma of the colon.

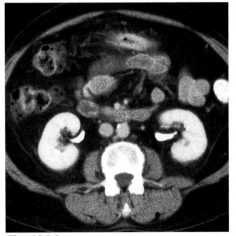

Fig. 134.3a

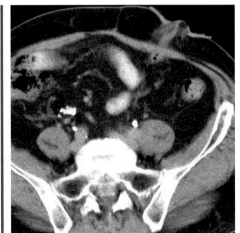

Fig. 134.4a

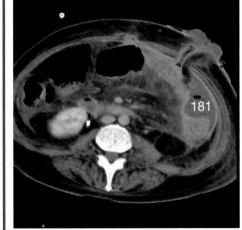

Fig. 134.5

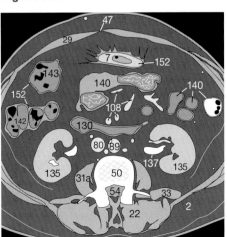

Fig. 134.3b

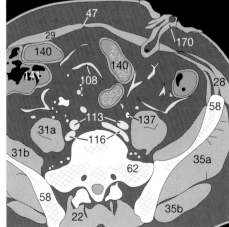

Fig. 134.4b

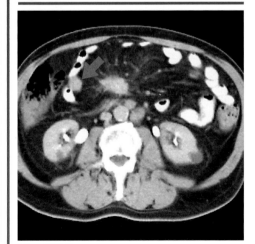

Fig. 134.6

Ileus

Horizontal air–fluid levels (⬇ ⬇) and atonic, dilated bowel loops **(140)** are typical features of ileus. If dilatation is recognized in the topogram **(Fig. 135.1)** or in an overview of the abdomen, an ileus must be suspected. If only the small intestine **(Fig. 135.2)** is involved, the most likely cause is a mechanical obstruction due to adhesions. A gallstone may cause obstruction of the small bowel (gallstone ileus). This follows cholecystitis with the formation of a cholecystoenteral fistula and the passage of a gallstone into the bowel. The gallstone may obstruct the narrower caliber of the distal ileum (**167** in **Fig. 135.3**).

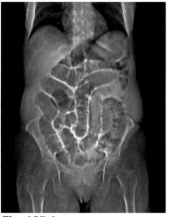

Fig. 135.1

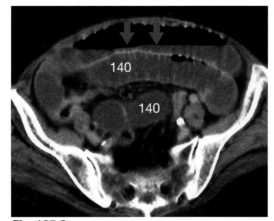

Fig. 135.2

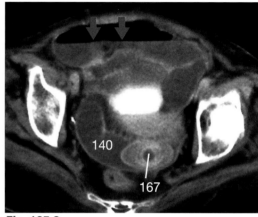

Fig. 135.3

Mechanical obstruction of the colon leads to similar air–fluid levels and dilatation (⬇ ⬇ in **Fig. 135.4**). When looking for the cause of an ileus, the entire colon must be examined for obstructing or constricting tumors or focal inflammation.

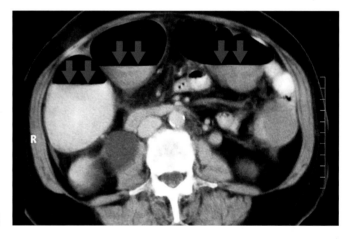

Fig. 135.4

Test Yourself!   Exercise 29:

Are there any suspicious findings other than the colic ileus in **Figure 135.4**? Does the image remind you of others in the manual? Make the most of the figures by returning to previous chapters, covering the text and identifying as many structures as possible. You will improve your learning efficiency by reviewing the images and diagrams and using the legends to make sure you got it right.

Space for notes and completing the exercise:

Aneurysms

Ectasia or aneurysms of the abdominal aorta **(89)** are usually the result of atherosclerotic disease **(174)** that leads to mural thrombosis **(173** in **Fig. 136.1)**. An aneurysm of the abdominal aorta is present if the diameter of the patent lumen has reached 3 cm or the outer diameter of the vessel measures more than 4 cm **(Fig. 136.2)**. Surgical intervention in asymptomatic patients is usually considered when the dilatation has reached a diameter of 5 cm. The general condition of the patient and the rate at which dilatation is progressing must be considered. If the patent lumen is central and is surrounded by mural thrombosis **(173** in **Fig. 136.2)**, the risk of rupture and consequent hemorrhage is reduced.

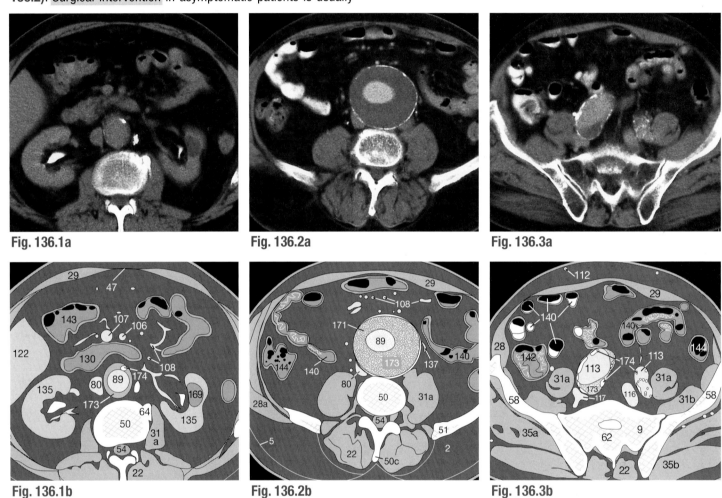

Fig. 136.1a

Fig. 136.2a

Fig. 136.3a

Fig. 136.1b

Fig. 136.2b

Fig. 136.3b

The risk of rupture is greater if the patent lumen is eccentric (↘ in **Fig. 136.4)** or if the cross-sectional shape of the vessel is very irregular. Dilatation in excess of 6 cm diameter also has a high risk of rupture. Surgical planning requires the determination of whether, and to what degree, the renal, mesenteric **(97)**, and iliac **(113)** arteries are involved by the aneurysm **(Fig. 136.3)**. Sudden pain may accompany rupture or dissection, which can extend from the thoracic to the abdominal aorta (cf. p. 103). Dynamic CM-enhanced CT will show the dissection flap **(172** in **Fig. 136.5)**.

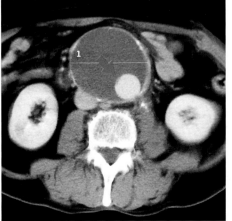

Fig. 136.4

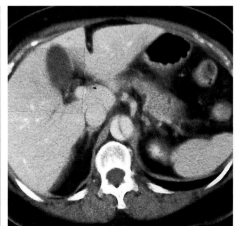

Fig. 136.5a

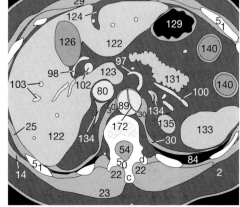

Fig. 136.5b

Venous Thromboses

In cases of thrombosis in a vein of the lower extremity (➡), venography does not always clearly show whether or not the thrombus extends into pelvic veins (Figs. 137.1a and 137.1b). The CM, which is injected into a superficial vein of the foot, is often diluted to such a degree that it becomes difficult to assess the lumen of the femoral/iliac veins (↘ in Fig. 137.1c). In such cases it is necessary to perform a CT with i.v. CM.

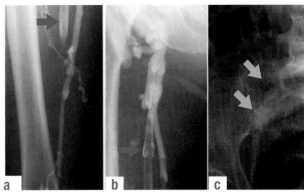

Fig. 137.1 a b c

The lumen of a vein containing a fresh thrombus (↘) is generally at least twice as large as normal (Fig. 137.2a). The segment containing the thrombus is either uniformly hypodense compared to the accompanying artery or it shows a hypodense filling defect, representing the thrombus itself. In the case illustrated on the right, the thrombus extended through the left common iliac vein (↗) to the caudal segment of the inferior vena cava (Fig. 137.2b) where it can be seen as a hypodense area (↑) surrounded by contrast-enhanced, flowing blood (Fig. 137.2c). CT slices must be continued cranially until the inferior vena cava no longer shows any signs of thrombus (↓ in Fig. 137.2d).

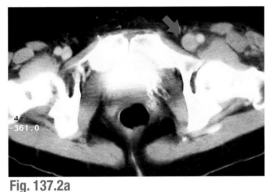

Fig. 137.2a

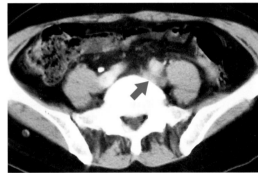

Fig. 137.2b

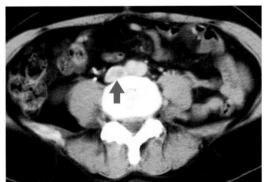

Fig. 137.2c

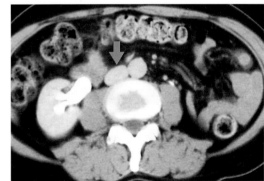

Fig. 137.2d

The injection of CM into a superficial foot vein opacifies satisfactorily only the ipsilateral leg, so it may be advisable to inject CM systemically through an arm vein in order to examine both sides of the pelvic venous system. If one side has become occluded, collaterals may develop (✳) via the prepubic network of veins (Figs. 137.3a and 137.3b). Such collaterals are known as a "Palma shunt" and these can also be surgically created if a thrombus in a deeper vein resists dissolution. You should be careful not to mistake an inguinal LN with physiologically hypodense hilar fat, "hilar fat sign" (✔ in Fig. 137.3c) for a partially thrombosed vein.

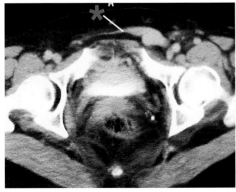

Fig. 137.3a

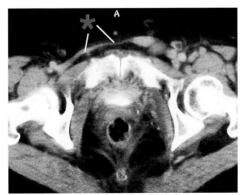

Fig. 137.3b

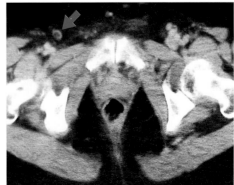

Fig. 137.3c

In order to avoid pulmonary embolism in cases of thrombosis (173) of the inferior vena cava (80 in Fig. 138.2), the patient must be immobilized until the thrombus has either become endothelialized or has responded to therapy and dissolved. Occasionally marked collateral circulation develops via the lumbar veins (121). Depending upon the individual patient and the size of the thrombus, the vessel may be surgically explored and thrombectomy performed. If thromboses are recurrent, an arterio-venous shunt may be indicated in order to avoid relapse. The success of a particular therapy may also be checked with venography or color-Doppler ultrasound.

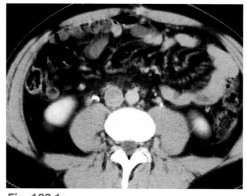

Fig. 138.1a

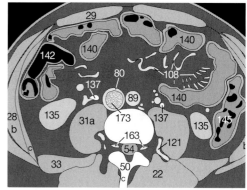

Fig. 138.1b

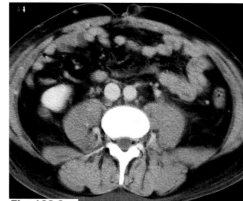

Fig. 138.2a

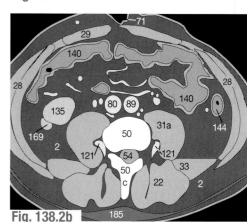

Fig. 138.2b

Enlarged Lymph Nodes

The density of LNs is approximately 50 HU, which corresponds to that of muscle. LNs with diameters below 1 cm are generally considered normal. Sizes between 1.0 and 1.5 cm are considered borderline and those that exceed 1.5 cm are abnormally enlarged. Sites of predilection for enlarged LNs are the retrocrural, mesenteric (↘), interaortico-caval (↖), and para-aortic spaces (cf. p. 81). **Figure 138.3** illustrates the case of a patient with chronic lymphatic leukemia.

It is essential to be familiar with the major paths of lymphatic drainage. The drainage of the gonads, for example, is directly to LNs at renal hilar level. LN metastases (↙ in Fig. 138.4) from a testicular tumor will be found in para-aortic nodes around the renal vessels but not in the iliac nodes, as would be expected with primary carcinomas of the urinary bladder, uterus, or prostate.

Conglomerate LN masses surrounding the aorta (89) and its major branches such as the celiac trunk (97) are a typical finding in cases of non-Hodgkin lymphoma (Fig. 138.5).

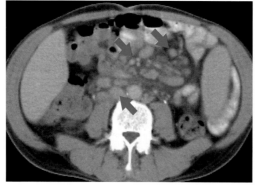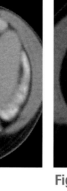

Fig. 138.3

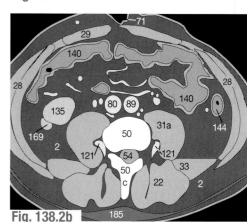

Fig. 138.4

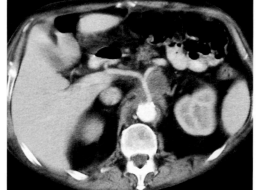

Fig. 138.5a

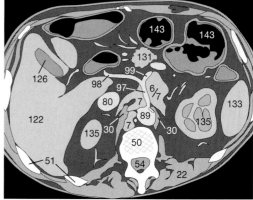

Fig. 138.5b

Normal Anatomy

The importance of examining bone windows during abdominal CTs has already been stressed on page 81. The marrow space of the iliac bones **(58)** and the sacrum **(62)** is normally homogeneous and the surfaces of the sacroiliac joints should be smooth and regular **(Fig. 139.1)**.

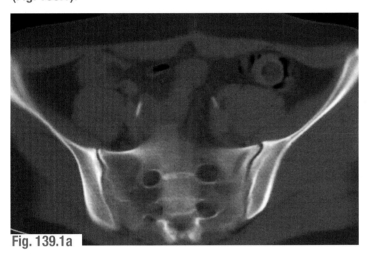

Fig. 139.1a

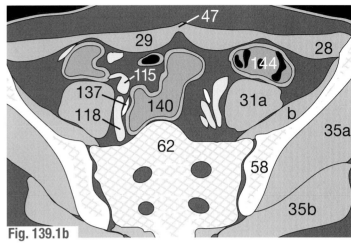

Fig. 139.1b

Metastases

Sclerotic bone metastases **(7)**, for example from a carcinoma of the prostate, are not always as evident as in **Figure 139.2a** and may vary in size and degree of calcification. Even small and poorly defined metastases should not be overlooked (✷ in **Fig. 134.2b**). They cannot routinely be recognized on soft-tissue windows.

Lytic metastases **(7)**, which can be seen on soft-tissue windows

(Fig. 139.3a) only after they have reached considerable size, can be much more accurately detected on bone windows **(Fig. 139.3c)**. This case shows a metastatic disease of the right ilium **(58)** that has destroyed the trabeculae and much of the cortex. The erosion extends to the sacroiliac joint. See the following pages for further images of this patient.

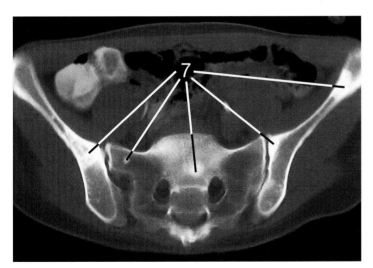

Fig. 139.2a

Fig. 139.2b

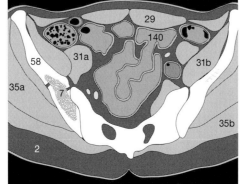

Fig. 139.3a

Fig. 139.3b

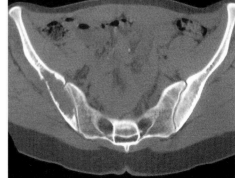

Fig. 139.3c

The mechanical integrity of a bone is suspect if any process involves its structure. Adjacent joint involvement must also be determined. MPRs (see p. 8) at various angles, for example sagittal or coronal, provide additional information. If necessary, 3D reconstructions can also be performed.

In the case shown on the previous page, (see **Fig. 139.3**) the question of stability is easily answered: the coronal MPR **(Fig. 140.1a)** shows that the trabeculae of the right iliac bone have been completely destroyed for approximately 10 cm (➡). The lesion extends from the acetabulum to the mid-point of the sacroiliac joint and has also destroyed much of the cortex. In several areas the cortex is disrupted (⬅). If you compare the bilateral sagittal reconstructions **(Figs. 140.1b and 1c)**, it is easy to see that there is acute risk of fracture.

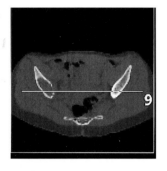

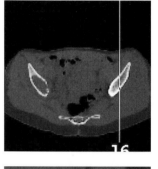

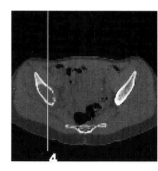

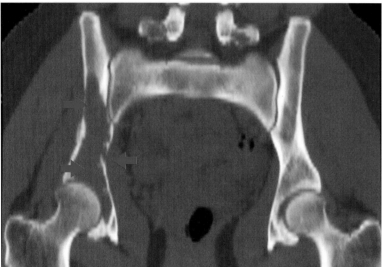

Fig. 140.1a

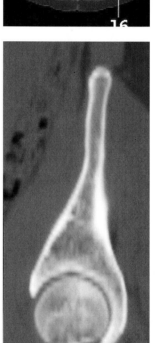

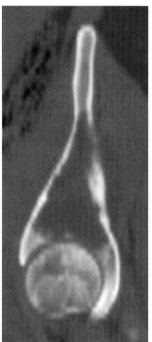

Fig. 140.1b   **Fig. 140.1c**

The 3D reconstruction of this pelvis **(Fig. 140.2)** does not add any more information, because it shows only the cortical disruption (🖢) as seen from the lateral perspective.

The degree to which the trabeculae and marrow have been destroyed cannot be seen in this reconstruction because the attenuation level was set to detect the cortical bone, and the deeper trabeculae are therefore covered.

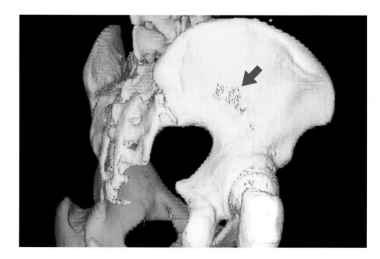

Fig. 140.2

Fractures

Bone windows should of course be used for the detection of fractures: hairline fractures and minimal dislocations cannot usually be recognized on soft-tissue windows.

It is also essential to give information on the precise fracture site and position of possible fragments for preoperative planning. In the case on the right, the fracture **(187)** of the femoral head **(66a)** is seen both in the axial plane **(Fig. 141.1)** and in the sagittal reconstruction **(Fig. 141.2)** (cf. p. 9).

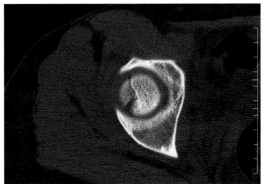

Fig. 141.1a

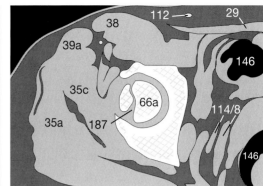

Fig. 141.1b

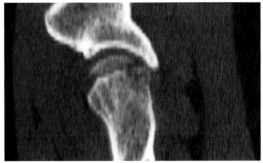

Fig. 141.2a

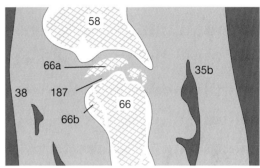

Fig. 141.2b

For joints such as the hip joint, it may be helpful to make an MPR in the oblique plane **(Figs. 141.3)**. The angle of reconstruction is shown in **Fig. 141.3a**. Be careful not to mistake the acetabular suture ( ) with the real ischial fracture ( )!

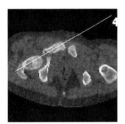

Fig. 141.3a

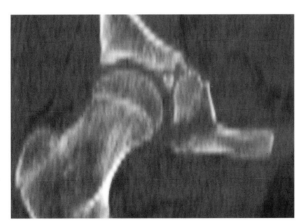

Fig. 141.3b

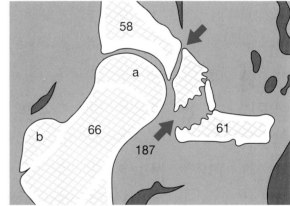

Fig. 141.3c

Another example of a fracture that may be mistaken for a suture is illustrated in **Figure 141.4**. The sutures ( ) are bilaterally symmetric, the fractures are not.

In this case several fragments of bone (⟷) are seen at the right iliopubic junction, but the right acetabulum is intact. Note also the asymmetry in the image which is caused by differences in the levels of the femoral heads. The patient had left acetabular dysplasia (cf. figures on p. 142).

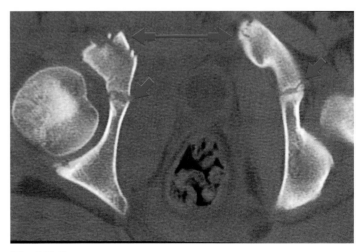

Fig. 141.4

Fragments are not always as obviously displaced nor is the fracture gap (🖢) as wide as in the case illustrated in **Figure 142.1**. Look for fine breaks (🡕) and discrete irregularities (🡠) in the cortical outline in order not to miss a fracture or a small fragment (**Fig. 142.2**).

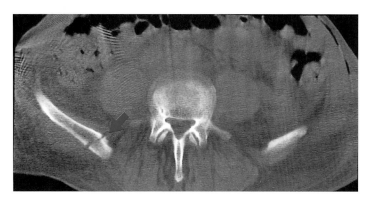

Fig. 142.1

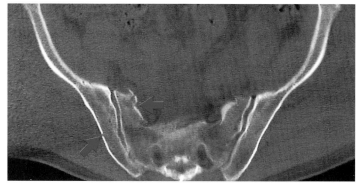

Fig. 142.2

Femoral Head Necrosis and Dysplasia of the Hip Joint

A fracture through the femoral head or even direct trauma to the hip joint may interrupt the blood supply to the head via the acetabular artery (see also **Figures 141.1** and **141.2**). Necrosis of the head makes it appear poorly defined (🖢) as seen in **Figure 142.3a** and causes shortening of the leg. An image obtained 2cm more cranially shows that a pseudoarthosis has developed in association with the right acetabular dysplasia (**Fig. 142.3b**). A 3D reconstruction gives an overview, but does not provide as much detail as a series of coronal MPRs (**Fig. 142.5b** with orientation in **Fig. 142.5a**).

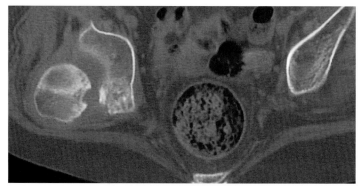

Fig. 142.3a

Fig. 142.3b

MPRs are often used for diagnostic purposes and in planning surgery of complex fractures. They contribute valuable additional information to the conventional axial images. SCT produces particularly accurate MPR images because disruptive step artifacts can be avoided if the patient is able to cooperate by holding his or her breath.

3D reconstructions, such as the one in **Figure 142.4**, yield impressive images, but are helpful only for specific problems such as plastic surgery. The amount of time and cost necessary to acquire and reconstruct 3D images are in most cases also very high.

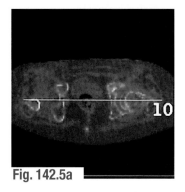

Fig. 142.4

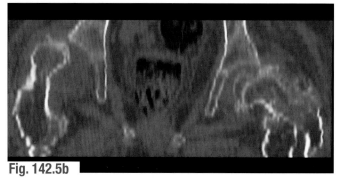

Fig. 142.5a   Fig. 142.5b

The images and questions on this page will again help you to check on how much you have understood; the questions become continually more difficult to answer. If you always remember the basic rules of CT reading, you will avoid jumping to the wrong conclusions. Don't look up the answers too soon!

Exercise 30:

What abnormality can you identify in **Figure 143.1**? Name as many blood vessels as you can!

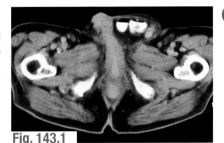

Fig. 143.1

Exercise 31:

Identify as many organs and blood vessels as possible in **Figure 143.2**. Look for any abnormalities.

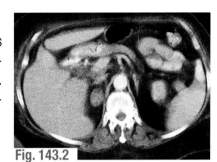

Fig. 143.2

Exercise 32:

What anatomic variation or abnormality do you recognize in **Figure 143.3**? Be sure you haven't missed anything.

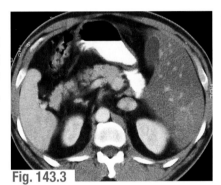

Fig. 143.3

Exercise 33:

"Do you smoke?" What abnormalities did you find in **Figure 143.4**?

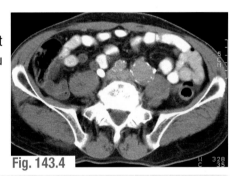

Fig. 143.4

Exercise 34:

It is easy to recognize the hepatic lesion in **Figure 143.5**. What is your DD?

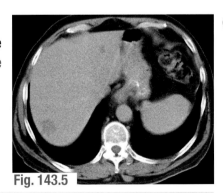

Fig. 143.5

Exercise 35:

Often abnormalities are not limited to one organ. What do your recognize in **Figure 143.6**?

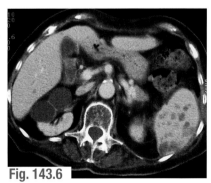

Fig. 143.6

The following questions may seem tricky, but you should be able to answer most of them if you go by the "rules of the book."

Exercise 36:
Describe the hepatic lesion in **Figure 144.1**. What steps did you take to ar-rive at your differential diagnosis? How would you proceed to verify it?

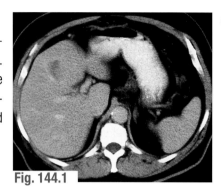

Fig. 144.1

Exercise 37:
Are the changes in **Figure 144.2** "normal," or do you suspect that they are pathologic findings?

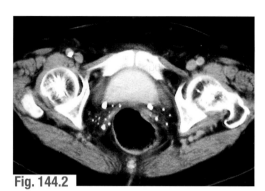

Fig. 144.2

Exercise 38:
Which of the two image levels on the right would you select for performing densitometric measurements of the kidney lesion? Why?

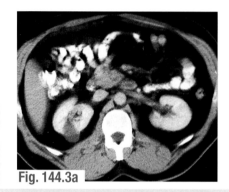

Fig. 144.3a

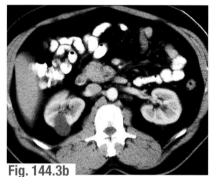

Fig. 144.3b

Exercise 39:
A patient is admitted for staging of a malignant melanoma (**Figure 144.4**). How far advanced is the lesion? What else would you do to obtain more information?

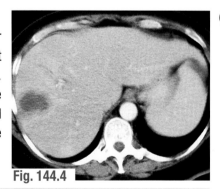

Fig. 144.4

Exercise 40:
A trauma patient could not be scanned in the prone position. What do you suspect in **Figure 144.5**, and what would you do to obtain more information?

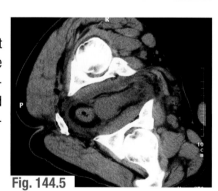

Fig. 144.5

Exercise 41:

A problem for those who already have some routine (**Figure 145.1**). How long did it take you to find two pathologic alterations and diagnose them accurately?

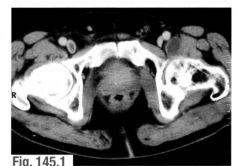
Fig. 145.1

Exercise 42:

Do you see anything abnormal in **Figure 145.2**? If so, what would you call it (the small figure indicates a structure filled with liquid)?

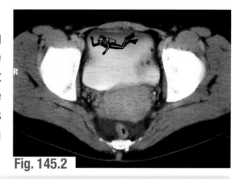
Fig. 145.2

Exercise 43:

At least three differential diagnoses should be considered for **Figure 145.3**. Which one is the most likely?

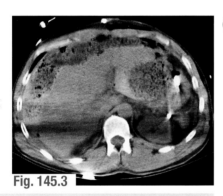
Fig. 145.3

Exercise 44:

In **Figure 145.4** there are also several possibilities to explain the obvious alteration. Are you able to find **all** possible lesions in an image of this kind?

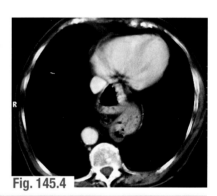
Fig. 145.4

Exercise 45:

What do you suspect is the case in **Figure 145.5**? What additional information do you need?

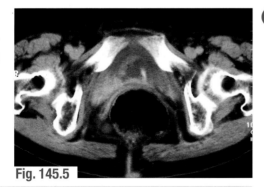
Fig. 145.5

Exercise 46:

This **Figure (145.6)** may contain several puzzles. Again, list the most likely diagnoses and then ask yourself what further information you need.

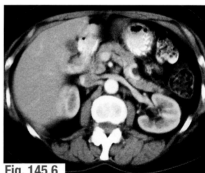
Fig. 145.6

The occipital condyles at the base of the skull articulate with the first vertebra, the atlas **(50a)**, which is the only vertebra to lack a body. The dens **(50b)** of the axis protrudes upward into the atlas and is held in place by the transverse ligament (★) **(Figs. 146.1** and **146.2)**. This ligament may be torn by a whiplash injury during road traffic accidents. The width of the space (←→) between the anterior arch of the atlas (★★ in **Figs. 146.1** and **146.2)** and the dens is also measured, as in conventional X-ray images **(Fig. 146.3)**. In adults it should not exceed 2 mm, in children 4 mm. The vertebral artery passes through the transverse foramen **(88)**.

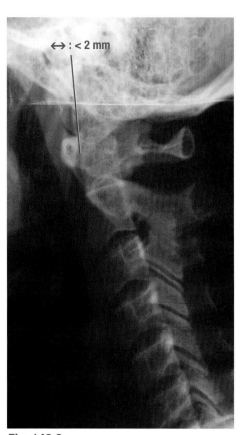

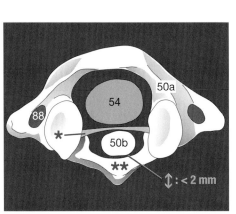

Fig. 146.1

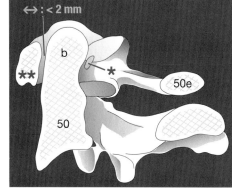

Fig. 146.2

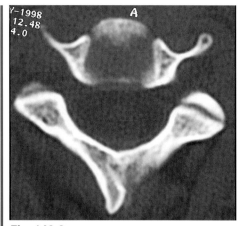

Fig. 146.3

The images below show normal anatomy at the level of the atlas **(Fig. 146.4)** and the body of the axis **(Fig. 146.5)**. The cartilage of an intervertebral disc **(50e** in **Fig. 146.6)**, will appear more homogeneous and hypodense than the typical pattern of trabeculae.

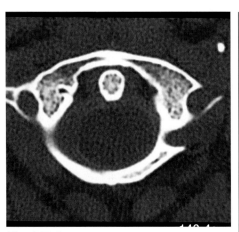

Fig. 146.4a

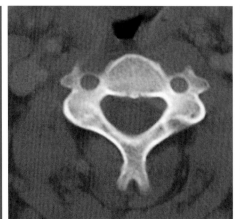

Fig. 146.5a

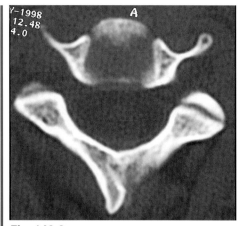

Fig. 146.6a

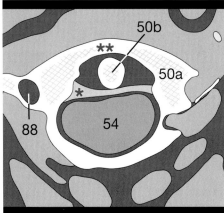

Fig. 146.4b

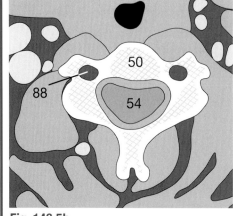

Fig. 146.5b

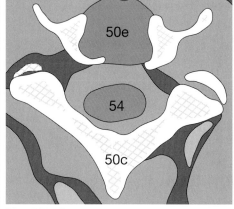

Fig. 146.6b

Cervical Disc Protrusion

A disc protrusion (prolaps of the nucleus pulposus) is demonstrated optimally in CT sections after myelography (CM in the SAS). The spinal cord is virtually isodense to CSF in unenhanced images, making it difficult to define the contours of the cord. After a myelogram, the CSF **(132)** will appear hyperdense to the cord **(54)** as well as to a disc.

Normally the CSF uniformly surrounds the cervical cord **(Fig. 147.1)**. A disc prolapse **(7)**, however, protruding into the CSF space can be seen because it is hypodense to the opacified CSF. The gap between the cord **(54)** and vertebral body **(50)** is filled in. Did you recognize the pyriform fossa **(172)**, the hyoid bone **(159)**, the thyroid cartilage **(169)**, and the cricoid cartilage **(167)**?

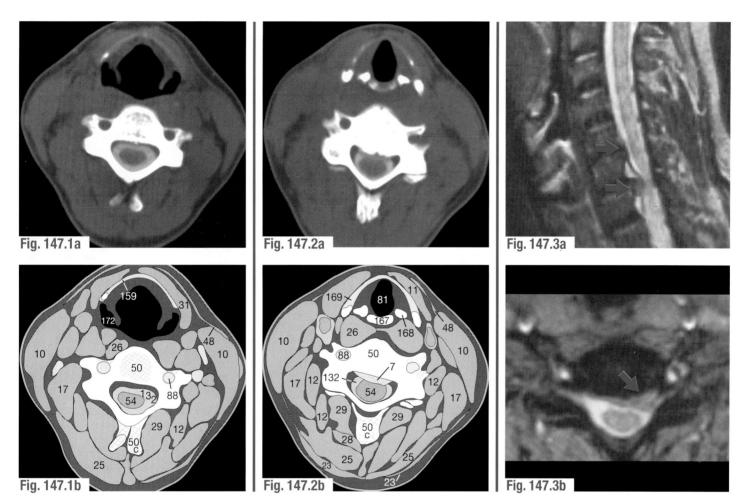

Fig. 147.1a

Fig. 147.2a

Fig. 147.3a

Fig. 147.1b

Fig. 147.2b

Fig. 147.3b

A disc prolapse will be seen even more clearly in an MR image. The sagittal T_2-weighted image in **Figure 147.3a** shows the extent of protrusions at two disk spaces. The disk protrudes into the hyperintense CSF space (➡) in front of the cord. The axial T_2-weighted image **(Fig. 147.3b)** shows that the prolapse extends to the left and has caused stenosis of the intervertebral foramen (➘).

Cervical Spine Fractures

It is especially important to look for fractures of the cervical spine or for torn ligaments after trauma so that damage to the cord is avoided if the patient needs to be moved or transported. **Figures** 147.4a through c show a coronal MPR in which the right occipital condyle **(160)** is fractured **(188)** but the dens **(50b)** is still in normal position.

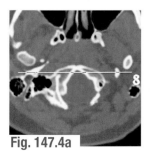

Fig. 147.4a

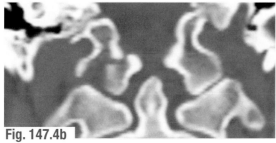

Fig. 147.4b

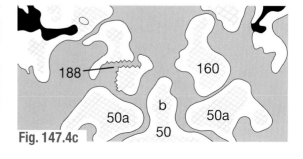

Fig. 147.4c

The thoracic vertebrae articulate with each other at their superior and inferior articular facets **(50d)** and with the ribs **(51)** at the inferior and superior costal facets and the transverse processes **(50f)**. **Figure 148.1** shows a normal thoracic image: the contours of the cortical bone are smooth and the trabeculae have a homogeneous pattern.

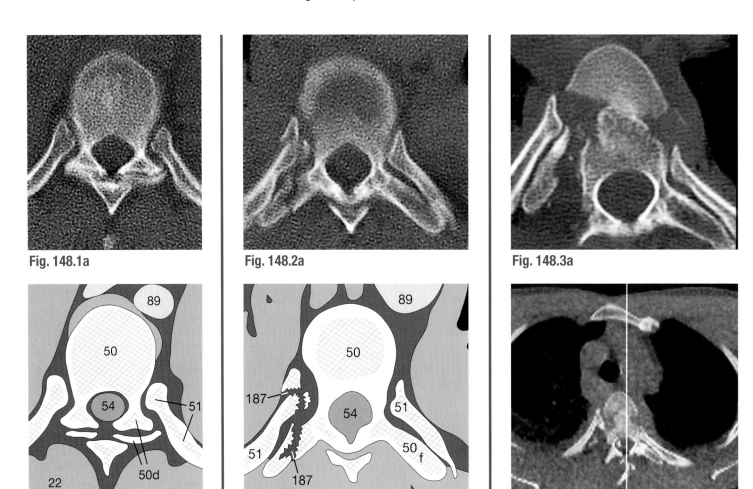

Fig. 148.1a

Fig. 148.2a

Fig. 148.3a

Fig. 148.1b

Fig. 148.2b

Fig. 148.3b

Fractures of the Thoracic Spine

Displaced fragments are identified by virtue of the fracture lines **(187)** and are best seen on bone windows. In **Figure 148.2** both the transverse process **(50f)** and the corresponding rib **(51)** are fractured. In complex fracture dislocations **(Figs. 148.3)** torsion or shearing may cause compression or complete dislocation of the spine as a whole **(Figs. 148.3a,e)**. The axial image in **Figure** 148.3a shows two vertebrae (✎) at one level; the topogram in 148.3b indicates the position of the sagittal MPR shown in **Figure** 148.3e. The MPR gives a more precise picture of the fracture and the fragments than the oblique anterior and oblique posterior 3D views in **Figures 148.3c** and **d**.

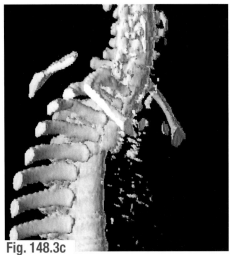

Fig. 148.3c

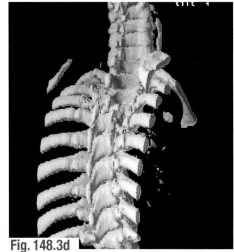

Fig. 148.3d

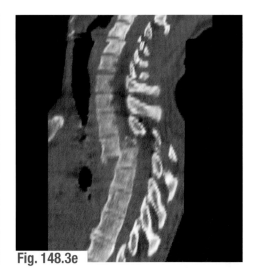

Fig. 148.3e

The transverse processes **(50f)** of the lumbar vertebrae are occasionally called costal processes. Lumbar vertebrae have much larger bodies **(50)** than thoracic vertebrae and the angle of their intervertebral joints **(50d)** is smaller. Lumbar spinous processes do not extend as far caudally as the thoracic ones. Images of the normal lumbar spine usually show well-defined cortical bone and homogeneous trabeculae. At the level of a disk **(Fig. 149.2)**, the hypodense cartilage **(50e)** may seem irregularly surrounded by bone: this is an oblique partial volume effect in which parts of an adjacent body **(50)** are included with the disk. The ligamenta flava (✶) extend from one lamina to the next and can sometimes be seen behind the cord **(Fig. 149.1a)**.

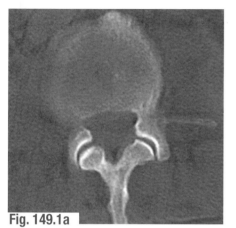

Fig. 149.1a

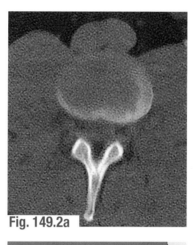

Fig. 149.2a

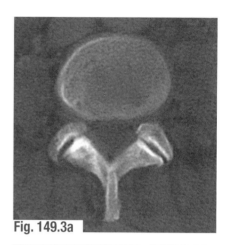

Fig. 149.3a

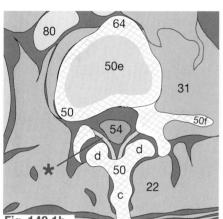

Fig. 149.1b

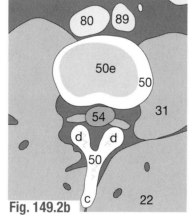

Fig. 149.2b

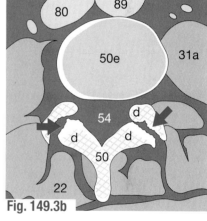

Fig. 149.3b

Degenerative change of the vertebrae can be seen in the facet joints **(50d)** **(Fig. 149.3)**. There is increased subchondral sclerosis (➡, ⬊) indicative of arthrosis of the joint.

Lumbar Disk Prolapse

As with cervical disk protrusions (see p. 147), it is important to establish whether the nucleus pulposus has protruded through the posterior longitudinal ligament. This ligament is applied to the posterior borders of the vertebral bodies and disks. Disk material that has penetrated the posterior longitudinal ligament and become detached from the disk is referred to as a sequestration (✶✶). This can narrow the spinal canal or a lateral recess **(Fig. 149.4)**. These structures are not well demonstrated on soft-tissue windows **(Fig. 149.4a)** because of their high density, but are clearly seen on bone windows **(Fig. 149.4b)**. A T$_2$-weighted MR image **(Fig. 149.5)** shows the extent of the prolapse: the abnormal disk (➡) is thinner, is desiccated (shows a lower signal level [darker]), and the extruded material (⬊) impinges on the theca.

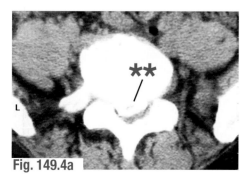

Fig. 149.4a

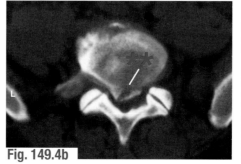

Fig. 149.4b

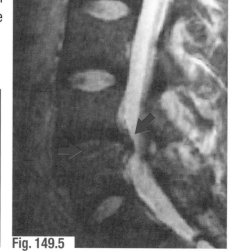

Fig. 149.5

Fractures

In conventional x-rays it is often difficult to see the fracture of a lumbar transverse process **(50f)** if the fragment is not or only minimally dislocated **(187)**. In CT sections, however, a fracture can be clearly demonstrated **(Fig. 150.1)**. **Figure 150.2** illustrates a case in which the spinous process **(50c)** was fractured. An arthrosis may develop if a fracture has involved a joint **(Fig. 150.3)**. There are fractures of both the superior and the inferior articular processes **(50d)**.

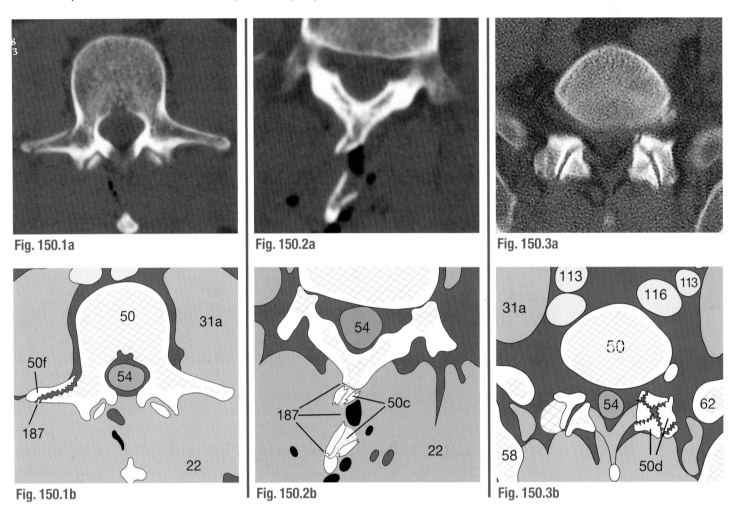

Fig. 150.1a

Fig. 150.2a

Fig. 150.3a

Fig. 150.1b

Fig. 150.2b

Fig. 150.3b

Older fractures do not show a well-defined fracture line **(187)**. Increased sclerosis and new bone often efface the fracture line or a pseudarthrosis may develop. In the case shown in **Figure 150.4** the fractured pedicle has developed a pseudarthosis. In conventional x-rays, increased sclerosis following a fracture is often difficult to differentiate from that resulting from degenerative disease.

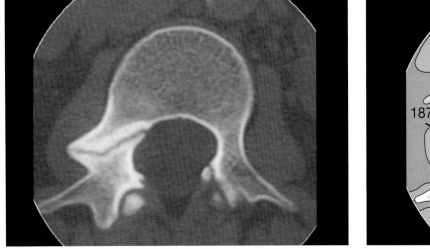

Fig. 150.4a

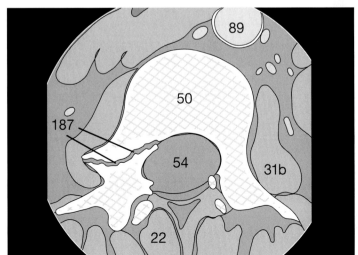

Fig. 150.4b

Tumors and Metastases

Not all bone lesions originate within the bone. Malignant tumors of paravertebral tissues can also invade the bones.

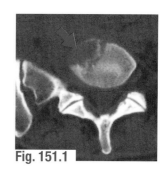

Figure 151.1 shows an osteolytic lesion (⬋) in the body of a lumbar vertebra in a patient with carcinoma of the cervix. On soft-tissue windows **(Fig. 151.2)** there is a paravertebral metastasis **(7)** which has surrounded the bifurcation of the common iliac artery **(114/5)** and has infiltrated the right anterolateral aspect of the vertebral body.

Fig. 151.1

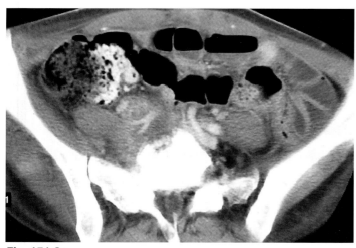

Fig. 151.2a

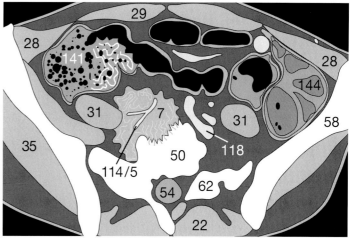

Fig. 151.2b

MPRs in the coronal **(Figs. 151.3a and b)** and sagittal **(Figs. 151.4a and b)** planes show the extent to which the bone has been eroded and that there is risk of fracture. As in **Figure 140.2**, the 3D reconstructions **(Figs. 151.5a and b)** clearly show the lesion from anterior and lateral perspectives, but not the degree to which the interior trabeculae have been destroyed.

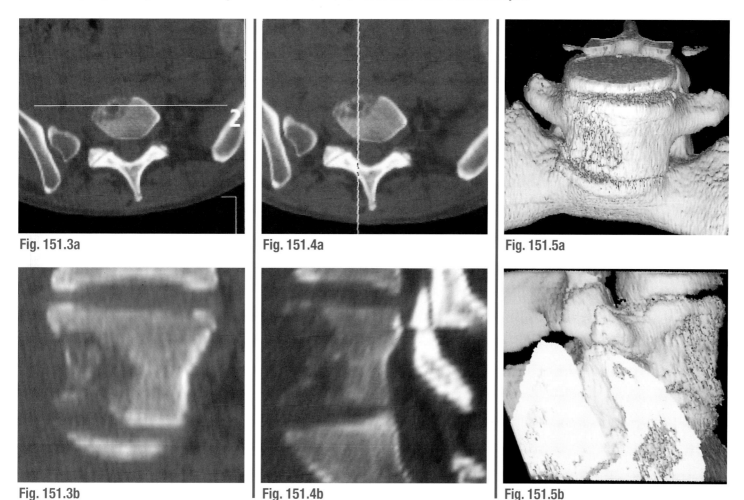

Fig. 151.3a

Fig. 151.4a

Fig. 151.5a

Fig. 151.3b

Fig. 151.4b

Fig. 151.5b

Infection

Abscesses in the paravertebral soft tissues or infective or inflammatory arthritides **(181)** in the small joints of the spine may lead to diskitis that ultimately destroys the intervertebral disk **(Fig. 152.1)**. An advanced abscess can be detected on soft-tissue windows **(Fig. 152.1a)** as an area of heterogeneous density surrounded by a hyperdense enhancing rim representing reactive hyperperfusion. On bone windows **(Fig. 152.1c)** only small remnants of bone belonging to the vertebral body are present and some are displaced.

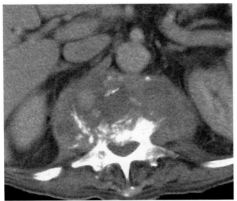

Fig. 152.1a

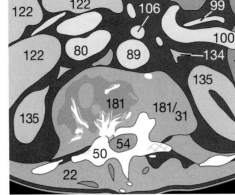

Fig. 152.1b

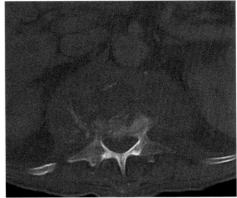

Fig. 152.1c

Methods of Stabilization

If therapeutic measures such as chemotherapy, antibiotics, and/or surgery have been effective in the treatment of a metastasis or infection, it is possible to stabilize the spine by inserting bone prosthetic material **(Fig. 152.2a, b)**. The choice of material depends upon the size of the defect and upon other individual factors. In follow-up examinations these materials may cause considerable image artifacts because of their high relative density.

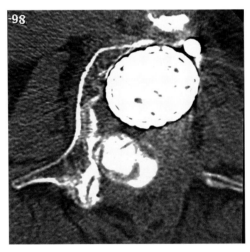

Fig. 152.2a

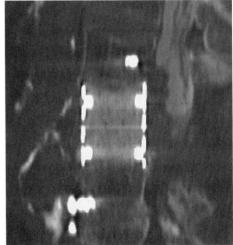

Fig. 152.2b

Space for additional notes:

The anterior muscles of the thigh include the sartorius muscle (38), and the four components of the quadriceps muscle (39). The most anterior is the rectus femoris (39a) and lateral to this is the vastus lateralis (39b). The vastus intermedius (39c) and vastus medialis (39d) form the anterolateral borders of the adductor canal. This contains the superficial femoral artery and vein (119/120). The adductor muscles comprise the superficially located gracilis muscle (38a), the adductor longus (44a), brevis (44b), and magnus (44c) muscles. The pectineus muscle (37) is only seen in the most caudal images of the pelvis.

The posterior muscles of the thigh extend the hip joint and flex the knee joint. The group consists of the long and short heads of the biceps femoris muscle (188), the semitendinosus (38b), and semimembranosus muscles (38c). In the proximal third of the thigh (Fig. 153.1) the hypointense tendon of the biceps muscle is adjacent to the sciatic nerve (162). In the distal third of the thigh (Fig. 153.3) the medial popliteal nerve (162a), which supplies the dorsal muscles, can be seen separate from the lateral popliteal nerve (162b). Note the close relationship of the profunda femoris artery and vein (119a/120a) to the femur (66) and the superficial position of the long saphenous vein (211a).

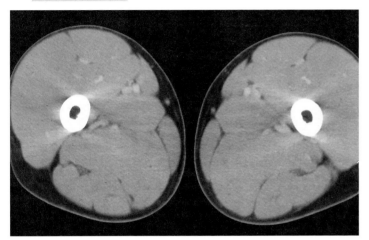

Fig. 153.1a

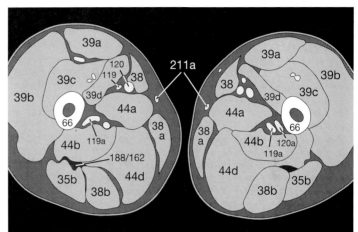

Fig. 153.1b

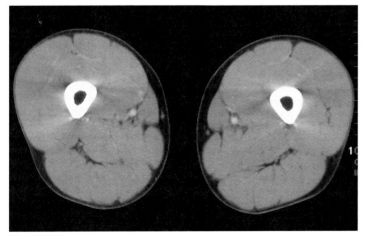

Fig. 153.2a

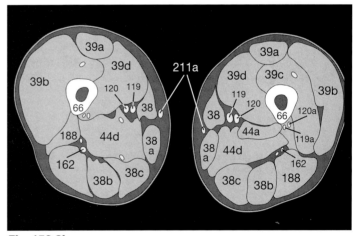

Fig. 153.2b

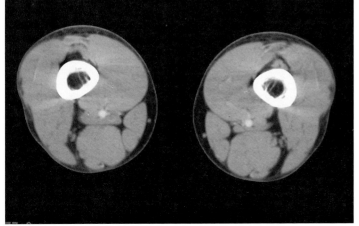

Fig. 153.3a

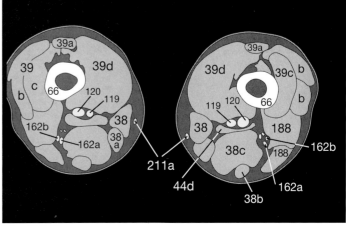

Fig. 153.3b

The popliteal artery **(209)** and vein **(210)**, formed cranial to the joint line, are demonstrated at the level of the patella **(191)** in the fossa between the femoral condyles **(66d)** **(Fig. 154.1)**. The tibial nerve **(162a)** lies directly posterior to the vein whereas the fibular (peroneal) nerve **(162b)** lies more laterally. The medial **(202a)** and lateral **(202b)** heads of the gastrocnemius muscle and the plantaris muscle **(203a)** can be seen posterior to the femoral condyles. The long saphenous vein **(211a)** lies medially in the subcutaneous fat covering the sartorius muscle **(38)**, and the biceps femoris muscle **(188)** lies laterally.

On the section just caudal to the patella **(Fig. 154.2)**, the patellar tendon **(191c)** can be identified, posterior to which is the infrapatellar fat pad **(2)**. Between the femoral condyles lie the cruciate ligaments **(191b)**.

Transverse sections such as these are frequently combined with coronal and sagittal MPRs (see also the images of a fracture on p. 161).

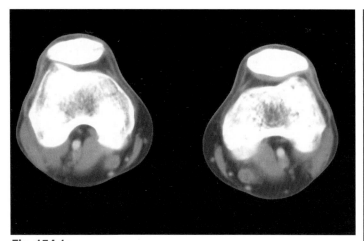

Fig. 154.1a

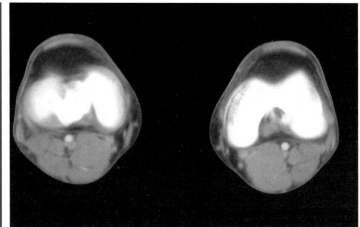

Fig. 154.2a

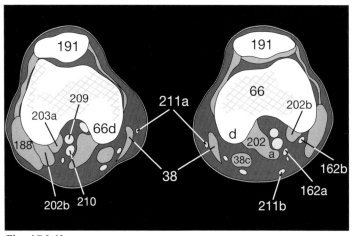

Fig. 154.1b

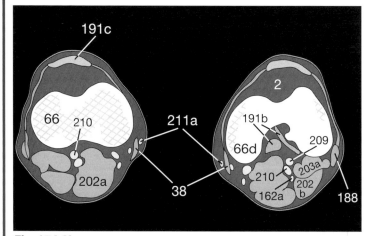

Fig. 154.2b

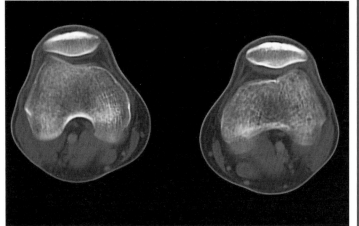

Fig. 154.1c

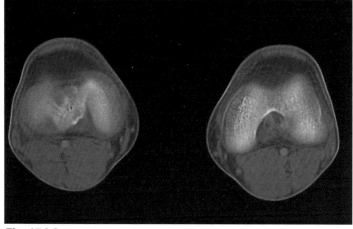

Fig. 154.2c

The muscles of the lower leg are separated into four compartments by the interosseus membrane between the tibia **(189)** and the fibula **(190)** and by the lateral and posterior intermuscular septa **(Figs. 155.1 to 155.3)**. The anterior compartment contains the tibialis anterior muscle **(199)**, the extensor hallucis longus muscle **(200a)** and the digitorum longus muscle **(200b)** next to the anterior tibial vessels **(212)**.

The lateral compartment contains the peroneus longus **(201a)** and brevis **(201b)** muscles next to the peroneal vessels **(214)**. In slender individuals who have no fat between the muscles, these vessels and the peroneal nerve are only poorly defined **(Fig. 155.2)**.

The flexor muscles can be separated into a superficial and a deep group. The superficial group encompasses the gastrocnemius muscle with medial **(202a)** and lateral **(202b)** heads, the soleus muscle **(203)** and the plantaris muscle **(203a)**. The deep group includes the tibialis posterior **(205)**, the flexor hallucis longus **(206a)**, and the flexor digitorum longus muscles **(206b)**. These muscles are particularly well defined in the distal third of the lower leg **(Fig. 155.3)**. The tibilalis posterior vessels **(213)** and the tibial nerve **(162a)** pass between the two flexor groups.

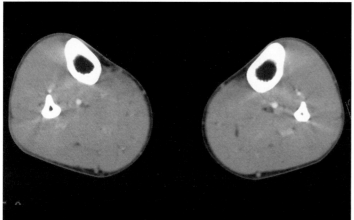

Fig. 155.1a

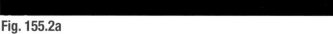

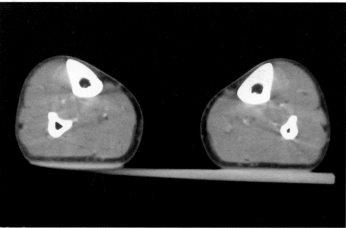

Fig. 155.2a

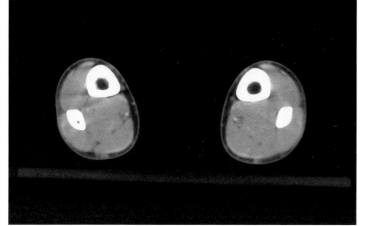

Fig. 155.3a

Fig. 155.1b

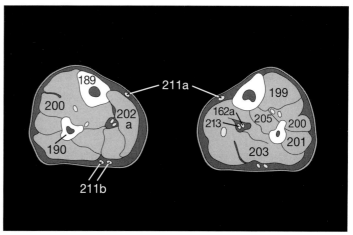

Fig. 155.2b

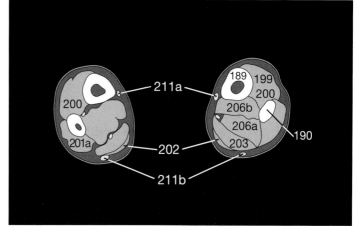

Fig. 155.3b

The following three pages show the normal anatomy of the foot on the bone window. You will find the number legends in the back fold-out.

The image series begins in a plane through the talus **(192)** just distal to the talocrural joint. **Figure 156.1** shows the distal end of the fibula or lateral malleolus **(190a)** as well as the upper part of the calcaneous **(193)**. In **Figure 156.2** the sustentaculum tali **(193a)** of the calcaneous is seen.

More distally, additional metatarsal bones are seen: the navicular bone **(194)** has begun to appear in **Figure 156.2**, but its joint with the talus is better assessed in **Figure 156.3**. The articular surfaces are normally smooth and the synovial space between the bones is of uniform width.

Compare these images of a normal foot with the images of fractures on pages 158 and 159.

The Achilles tendon **(215)**, which arises from both the soleus **(203)** and the gastrocnemius **(202)** muscles is seen posteriorly on these images.

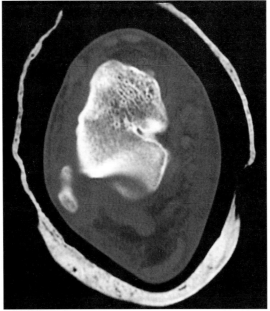

Fig. 156.1a

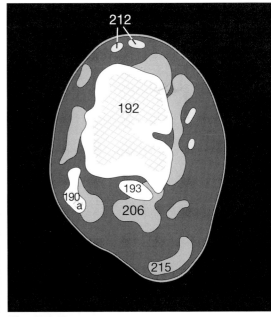

Fig. 156.1b

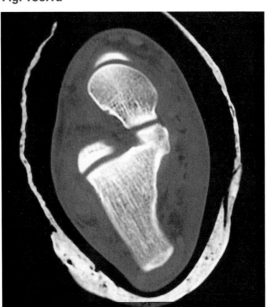

Fig. 156.2a

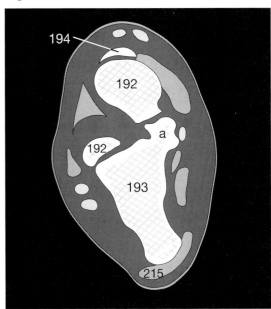

Fig. 156.2b

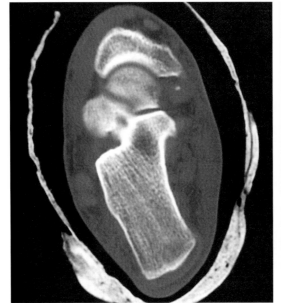

Fig. 156.3a

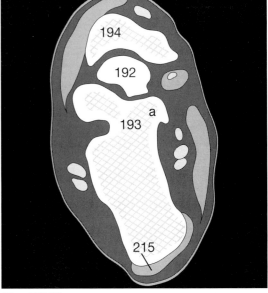

Fig. 156.3b

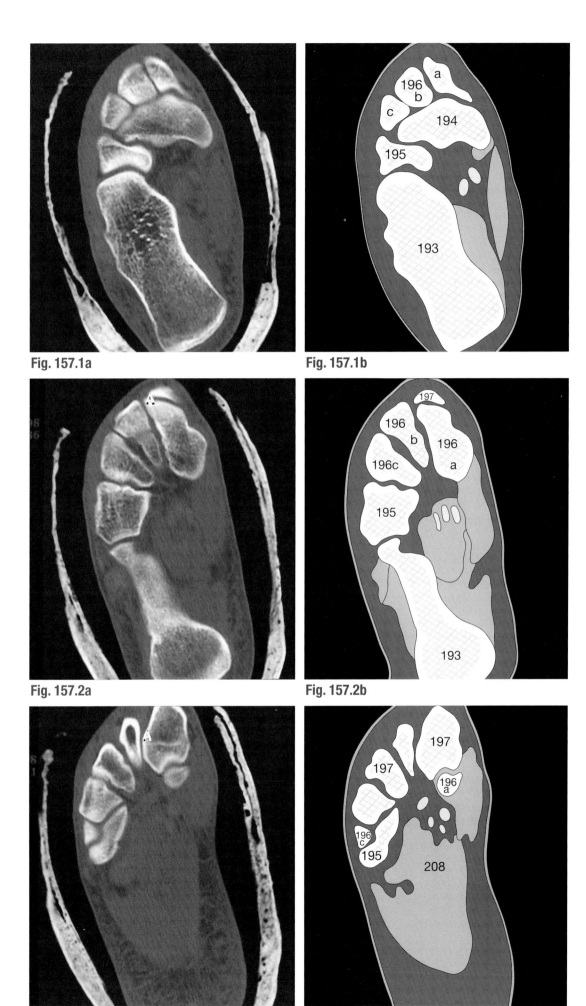

Fig. 157.1a

Fig. 157.1b

Fig. 157.2a

Fig. 157.2b

Fig. 157.3a

Fig. 157.3b

The cuboid bone **(195)** is seen on the lateral margin of the foot, between the calcaneus **(193)** and the navicular **(194)**. The lateral **(196c)**, intermediate **(196b)** and medial **(196a)** cuneiform bones lie anterior to the navicular **(Fig. 157.1)**.

The transition to the metatarsal bones **(197)** is not always well defined, due to partial volume effects, because the plane of the tarsometatarsal joints is at an oblique angle to the sections **(Fig. 157.2)**. The joints can be more clearly assessed in multiplanar reconstructions that take this obliquity into account (cf. **Fig. 158.1**).

The lumbrical and quadratus plantae muscles and the short flexor muscles of the foot **(208)** are seen just below the arch of the metatarsal bones. These muscles are only poorly defined in CT images **(Fig. 157.3)**.

Multiplanar reconstructions are very valuable for visualizing fractures of the foot. The lateral digital radiograph in **Figure 158.1a** indicates the angle of the image plane, parallel to the long axis of the

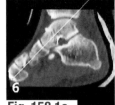

Fig. 158.1a

foot, seen in **Figure 158.1b**. This reconstructed image extends from the lateral **(190a)** and medial **(189a)** malleoli (at the lower edge of the image) through the talus **(192)** and the navicular **(194)** to the three cuneiform bones **(196a–c)**. Two of the metatarsal bones **(197)** are included in the section. Note that the surfaces of the joints are smooth and evenly spaced.

The sagittal image in **Figure 158.2b** was reconstructed slightly more laterally (see position in **158.2a**) so that the cuboid bone **(195)** is included. The short flexor muscles **(208)** and the plantar ligaments are seen below the arch of the foot. The Achilles tendon **(215)** is seen posteriorly.

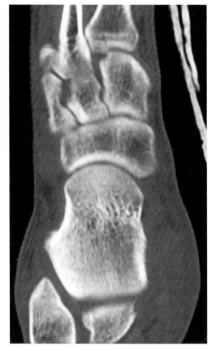

Fig. 158.1b

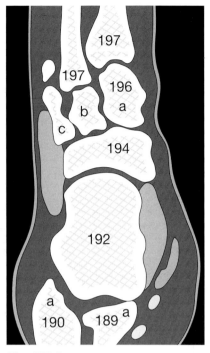

Fig. 158.1c

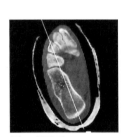

Fig. 158.2a

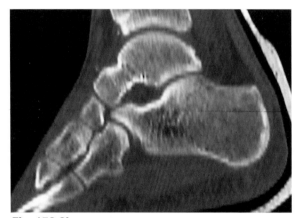

Fig. 158.2b

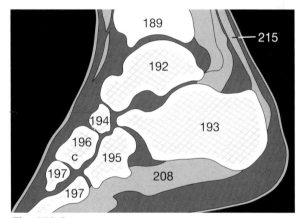

Fig. 158.2c

Diagnosis of Fractures

Typical signs of a fracture can be seen in the original axial plane **(Fig. 158.3a)**: irregularities in the cortical outline (⬇), displaced fragments (⬈) and a fracture line (⬅) in the calcaneous. The MPR in the coronal plane (indicated in **Fig. 158.3b**) shows that not only is the calcaneous (⬉) fractured, but there is a hairline fracture of the talus (➡) involving the ankle joint **(Fig. 158.3c)**.

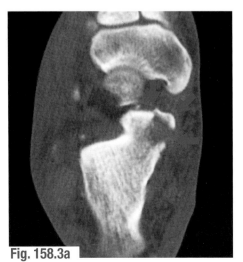

Fig. 158.3a

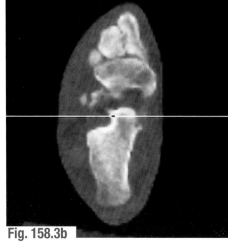

Fig. 158.3b

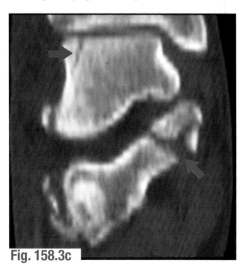

Fig. 158.3c

Fractures of the foot may initially escape detection in conventional x-rays if there is no major displacement of bone fragments. If the foot remains painful, a follow-up X-ray may show the fracture because fine hairline fractures can be seen when filled with hemorrhage. As an alternative, CT would show discrete fracture lines **(187)**, as for example of the talus **(192)** in **Figure 159.1**.

In chronic fractures, the displaced fragment (✱) has usually become rounded off **(Fig. 159.2)**. In this example it is obvious that there were actually two fragments because a second fracture line (⬇) is seen next to the main one **(187)**.

It is often difficult to treat comminuted fractures of the calcaneus **(193)**, incurred for example during a fall **(Fig. 159.3)** because there are many small displaced fragments. A stabile reconstruction of the arch of the foot may not be possible, resulting in a long period of sick leave.

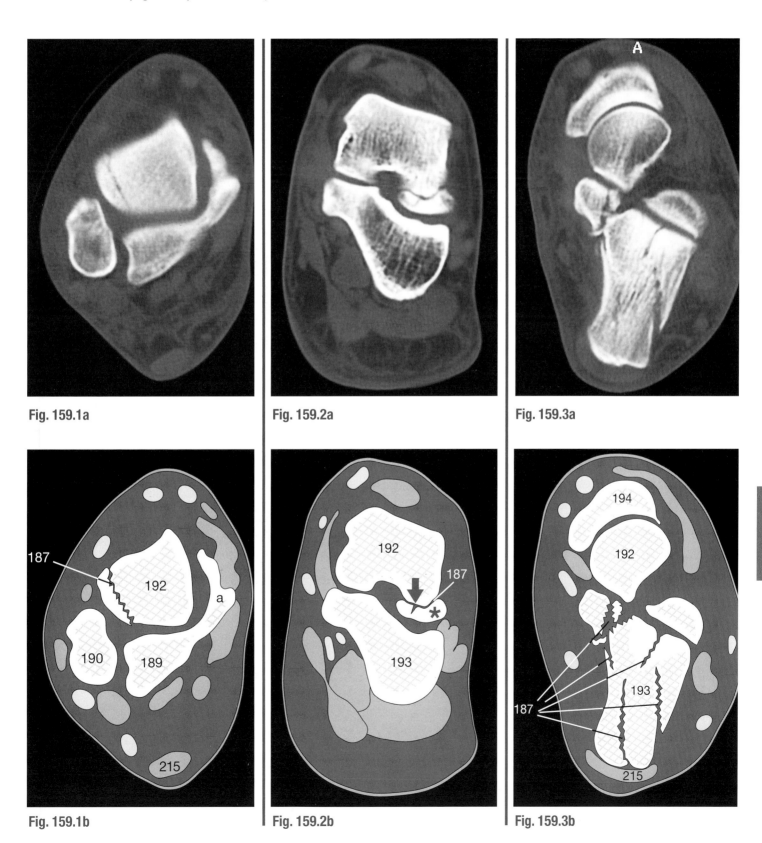

Fig. 159.1a

Fig. 159.2a

Fig. 159.3a

Fig. 159.1b

Fig. 159.2b

Fig. 159.3b

Infections

The assessment of fractures of long bones is generally the domain of conventional radiology. But CT examinations are helpful for locating displaced fragments and in the preoperative planning of comminuted fractures. Infections, however, are more accurately imaged by CT than conventional radiographs because bone destruction is more readily seen on bone windows **(Fig. 160. 1c)** and soft-tissue involvement **(178)** is documented on soft-tissue windows **(Fig. 160.1a)**. This patient had septic arthritis of the left hip joint with involvement of the acetabulum **(60)** and femoral head **(66a)**.

The abscess appears more clearly after contrast enhancement (cf. **Figs. 160.2a** and **160.2c**). The increased vascularity of the wall and the fluid within the abscess **(181)** are well demarcated from surrounding fat **(2)**. Adjacent muscles **(38, 39, 44)** are no longer individually defined because of edema (compare with the right leg). Gas **(4)** has been produced and is loculated in the adjacent tissues.

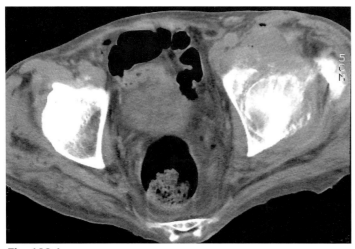

Fig. 160.1a

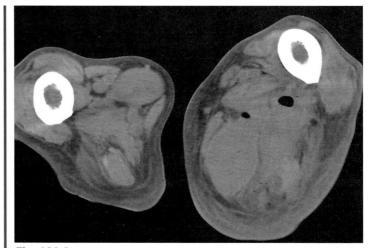

Fig. 160.2a

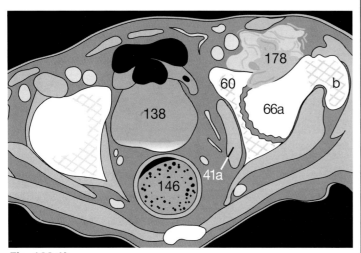

Fig. 160.1b

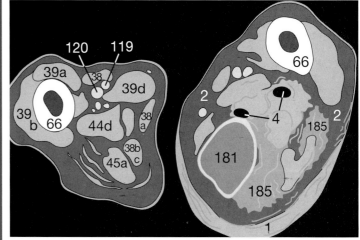

Fig. 160.2b

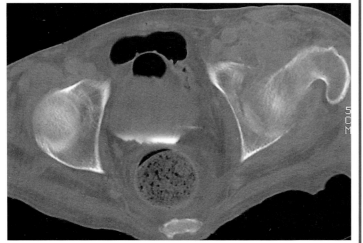

Fig. 160.1c

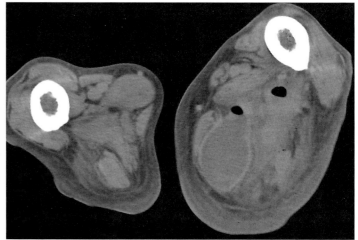

Fig. 160.2c

Fractures

If a fracture involves the knee joint, it is particularly important to reduce the fragments accurately to avoid joint surface incongruities that might lead to arthosis. In the case below, axial sections clearly show the lateral displacement of a large fragment (✒) of the tibia (**Figs. 161.1a** and **161.1b**). The coronal MPR (**Fig. 161.2b**, with level shown in **161.2a**) illustrates how much of the tibial plateau is affected.

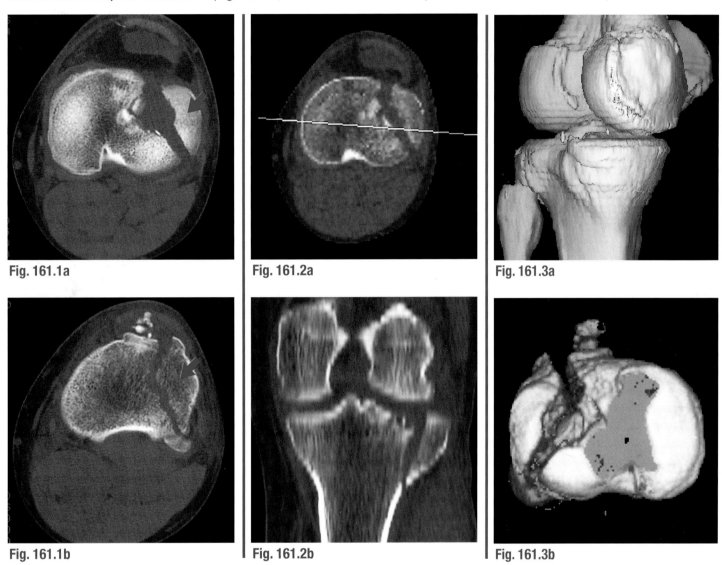

Fig. 161.1a   Fig. 161.2a   Fig. 161.3a

Fig. 161.1b   Fig. 161.2b   Fig. 161.3b

The 3D reconstruction seen from a posterolateral projection (**Fig. 161.3a**) is not very helpful, but the view from cranial (**Fig. 161.3b**) gives a good impression of the tibial plateau and the fracture line because the femoral condyles have been excluded.

Space for notes:

It is not always possible to determine the nature of a lesion from CT appearance and densitometry alone. In these cases needle biopsies may be carried out under ultrasound or CT guidance. The patient's platelet count and coagulation status must be checked and informed consent obtained.

In **Figure 161.1**, a mass in the caudate lobe (★) of the liver **(122)** is being biopsied. The close proximity of the hepatic artery and portal vein **(98/102)** and inferior vena cava **(80)** leave only a narrow path for the needle to approach from the right side **(Fig. 135.1a)**. Firstly the section on which the lesion appears largest is determined. The skin is cleaned and anesthetized with local anaestheic.

The needle is then inserted through the liver parenchyma toward the lesion. Slight changes in angle may be necessary **(Figs. 162.1b, 162.1c, and 162.1d)**. Distances can also be calculated during the procedure as seen in **Figure 162.1b**. After biopsy has been completed, an image is acquired to detect any hemorrhage. If a pneumothorax occurred following lung biopsy, expiratory images of the thorax are acquired to check for a tension pneumothorax.

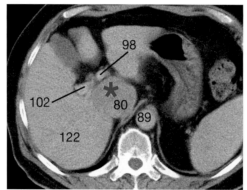

Fig. 162.1a

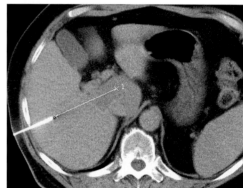

Fig. 162.1b

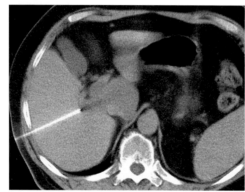

Fig. 162.1c

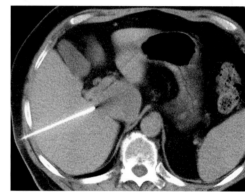

Fig. 162.1d

If there is a retroperitoneal lesion close to the spinal column, a biopsy may be carried out in the prone position. The orientation in **Figure 162.2** is therefore unusual and one must be careful not to confuse left with right, but the procedure is identical.

After selection of the optimal level (largest diameter of the lesion) and after skin cleaning and local anesthesia, the needle is inserted **(Fig. 162.2b)** and the biopsy taken. The material should be promptly prepared for cytology and histology.

The size and extent of a cutaneous fistula can often be more clearly assessed if CM is instilled through a tube **(Fig. 162.3)**. In this example the hip had become infected and an abscess filled the joint after prosthetic surgery.

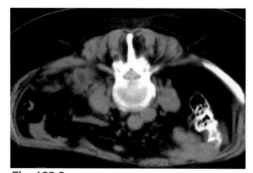

Fig. 162.2a

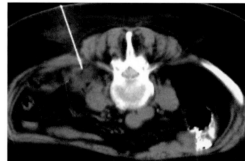

Fig. 162.2b

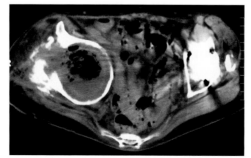

Fig. 162.3a

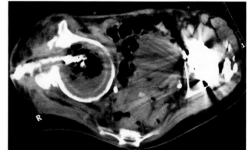

Fig. 162.3b

Recent developments in SCT techniques have shortened the time needed for data acquisition, allowing the acquisition of images during the different perfusion phases of a CM bolus. Biphasic and triphasic perfusion studies of the liver are well documented [17, 18, 21, 22, 35, 40]. Technical issues such as determining optimal CM flow, establishing the best start-delay times, or dividing CM injections with intervening pauses are still being discussed and are the subject of clinical research.

Flow

Some radiologists examine the liver at a flow rate of 3 to 6 ml/sec [36, 37, 38], but there is no significant difference in the detection of focal hepatic abnormalities using a reduced flow rate of only 2 ml/sec [21, 40]. Differences in flow rate are important for choosing the caliber and position of the i.v. line.

Pitch

Small lesions are detected more reliably when the pitch is low. The pitch represents the relationship between table speed/gantry rotation and d_S. For example, if both table speed and d_S in routine chest and abdominal CT are equal to 8 mm, then the pitch factor is 1.

In order to reduce radiation load, the table speed can be larger than the d_S. This will produce gaps in the volume data set that can only be avoided if the d_S is increased (see also the chapter on partial volume effects, p. 10). If effective d_S needs to be small, such as in neck CT, then a table speed of 5 mm with a d_S of 5 mm will also yield a pitch of 1.

If, for example in chest CTs, d_S is 10 mm and table speed 8 mm, the slices will overlap and the pitch will be 0.8.

Scan Delay

The optimal time point to begin data acquisition after i.v. injection of CM depends on both the clinical condition of each individual patient and the chosen flow rate. The scan delay should be longer for patients with cardiac failure, possibly twice as long as normal.

Suggested times on the following pages are for patients without any cardiac disease. Hardware applications detecting the arrival of the CM bolus have been developed so that the best enhancement images can be acquired.

Injection Protocol

The amount of CM used is kept at a minimum, not only for financial reasons, but also to avoid renal problems. It is therefore important to find a technique that produces clear definition of blood vessels with the least amount of CM. Many radiologists inject i.v. CM at constant flow rates, others have demonstrated that definition is better when biphasic injection technique is used, for example in neck CT. Injection methods will improve as more radiologists routinely use SCT. So far, experience has shown that using pressure injectors leads to more homogeneous opacification and more reliable results than hand injections.

Trial Injection

If a pump injector is used, the i.v. catheter should first be checked manually in order to insure proper position and to determine the volume capacity of the vein. The automated flow rate is then adjusted to this capacity to avoid vascular damage or extravasation.

For readers interested in further information, references 34 and 39 are suggested.

Space for notes:

The following protocols were developed from information in the literature and from our own experience. The terms in the blue headers are discussed on the previous page (see also p. 9). The amounts of nonionic CM are given for an average patient of 75 kg b.w. and are calculated for CM with an iodine content of 300 mg/ml. Dosage may need to be adjusted depending on b.w. (at an average of approximately 1.2 ml CM/kg b.w.) and the state of the patient's circulatory system (changes in scan delay). For example, if a patient weighs 90 kg, the total amount of CM for a CCT would be increased to 110 mg.

Head: sequential acquisition (caudal to cranial)

Slice (mm)	Advance (mm)	Pitch	Scan delay (sec)	Total CM (ml)	Flow (ml/sec)	Comments
2	4	2	60	90	2.0	base of skull
8	8	1				above petrosal bone

Neck: dynamic sequential acquisition (cranial to caudal)

Slice (mm)	Advance (mm)	Pitch	Scan delay (sec)	Total CM (ml)	Flow (ml/sec)	Comments
5	5	1	30	100-120	2.0	no swallowing!

Neck: spiral CT (cranial to caudal)

Slice (mm)	Advance (mm)	Pitch	Scan delay (sec)	Total CM (ml)	Flow (ml/sec)	Comments
5	5	1	40	90-100		
				first 50	2.0	1st bolus
						5 sec pause
				then 40-50	1.5	2nd bolus

Thorax: sequential acquisition (caudal to cranial)

Slice (mm)	Advance (mm)	Pitch	Scan delay (sec)	Total CM (ml)	Flow (ml/sec)	Comments
8	8	1	40	120		
				first 60	2.0	no pause
				then 60	1.5	

Thorax: Spiral CT (caudal to cranial)

Slice (mm)	Advance (mm)	Pitch	Scan delay (sec)	Total CM (ml)	Flow (ml/sec)	Comments
10	8	0.8	50	100	2.0	(2-3 spirals)

Note:

If thorax CT is carried out in the craniocaudal direction, the start delay must be reduced to approximately 15 seconds; beam-hardening effects close to the subclavian vein are likely (see also p. 21).

Aorta: thorax–abdomen sequential acquisition (cranial to caudal)

Slice (mm)	Advance (mm)	Pitch	Scan delay (sec)	Total CM (ml)	Flow (ml/sec)	Comments
10	10	1	15	160		no pause
				first 100	2.0	
				then 60	1.5	

Aorta: thorax–abdomen spiral CT (cranial to caudal)

Slice (mm)	Advance (mm)	Pitch	Scan delay (sec)	Total CM (ml)	Flow (ml/sec)	Comments
5	10	2	20	140		
				first 80	3.0	0-20 sec pause
				then 60	2.5	(3-4 spirals)

Abdomen: sequential acquisition (cranial to caudal) (after unenhanced CT of liver)

Slice (mm)	Advance (mm)	Pitch	Scan delay (sec)	Total CM (ml)	Flow (ml/sec)	Comments
10	10	1	40	100-140	2.0	

Abdomen: spiral CT (biphasic liver imaging in two spiral acquisitions)

(First spiral from caudal to cranial, second spiral from cranial to caudal, followed by sequential imaging more caudally)

Slice (mm)	Advance (mm)	Pitch	Scan delay (sec)	Total CM (ml)	Flow (ml/sec)	Comments
10	8	0.8	15	100-120	2.1	see below

Note:

Each spiral should take no longer than 20 seconds (the patient must hold his or her breath!). During pauses (5 sec) the patient can breathe and the tube can cool. The change in direction between the first and the second spiral saves time because the second spiral can begin where the first finished: at the level of the diaphragm.

Image acquisition caudal to the liver should not commence too quickly after the second spiral because of incomplete renal enhancement. It is therefore useful to use the sequential mode for image acquisition of the kidneys and pelvis instead of a third spiral. Alternatively, 20 ml of CM can be injected 5 minutes before CT so that ureter and bladder are opacified during SCT of the liver. The abdomen can then be rapidly examined in three to four spirals. This technique does not affect the detection of hepatic abnormalities during the arterial phase spiral.

Pancreas: sequential or spiral CT (cranial to caudal)

Slice (mm)	Advance (mm)	Pitch	Scan delay (sec)	Total CM (ml)	Flow (ml/sec)	Comments
5	5	1	40	90-100	2.0	see below

Note:

Water, instead of oral CM, may be used to outline the lumen of the duodenum. In CT for pancreatitis, the start delay should be increased to about 60-70 seconds so that the splenic vein and the branches of the portal vein are also opacified. The entire liver and pelvis should be included in the examination in order to detect any complications such as cholestasis, ascites, and necrosis. The d_S (10 mm) and table speed are the same as in other abdominal CT protocols.

The exercises and solutions have been numbered consecutively. Some of the exercises have several different correct solutions. If the exercises can be solved simply by referring to the chapters in the book, I have indicated where you will find the necessary information.

After you have completed the exercises, compare your score and results with those of your colleagues. The score on the right gives you an impression of the degree of difficulty. Enjoy the challenge!

Solution to exercise 1 (p. 30):   9 Points

You will find the sequence for interpreting CCTs on page 24. Each step gives you ½ point with 3 extra points for the correct sequence, which adds up to 9.

Solution to exercise 2 (p. 43):   9 Points

	Level	Width	Gray scale	
Lung/pleural window	- 200 HU	2000 HU	-1200 to + 800 HU	3
Bone window	+300 HU	1500 HU	- 450 to +1050 HU	3
Soft-tissue window	+ 50 HU	350 HU	- 125 to + 225 HU	3

Solution to exercise 3 (p. 43):   10 Points

a)	Barium sulfate	Routine for abdominal/pelvic CT if there are no contraindications	30 min before CT of upper abdomen 60 min before full abdominal CT	4
b)	Gastrografin	Water soluble, but expensive; if perforation ileus or fistulas are suspected; prior to surgery	20 min before CT of upper abdomen 45 min before full abdominal CT	4
				1

No oral CM shortly after surgery for an ileal conduit!   1

Solution to exercise 4 (p. 43):   6 Points

a)	Renal failure (creatinine, possibly creatinine clearance, function following kidney transplant or nephrectomy)	2
b)	Hyperthyroidism (clinical signs? if yes, hormone status, possibly thyroid ultrasound and scintigraphy)	2
c)	Allergy to CM (has CM-containing iodine already been injected? Are there any known previous allergic reactions?)	2

Solution to exercise 5 (p. 43):   2 Points

Tubular and nodular structures can be differentiated by comparing a series of images.

Solution to exercise 6 (p. 43):   3 Points

Vessels in which beam-hardening artifacts occur because of CM inflow are the superior vena cava, inferior vena cava, and the subclavian vein.

Solution to exercise 7 (p. 46):   3 Points

Fractures, inflammatory processes, and tumors or metastases can cause swelling of mucous membranes and retention of fluids in the mastoid sinuses and middle ear; these are normally filled with air.

Solution to exercise 8 (p. 55):   18 Points

This image requires careful study. You will discover several types of intracranial hemorrhage and the complications resulting from them.

- Bruising of the left frontoparietal soft tissues (extracranial, indicative of trauma to the head)   1
- Subdural hematoma over the right hemisphere extending to occipital levels (hyperdense)   2
- Edema in the right frontoparietal areas, possibly accompanied by an epidural hematoma   2
- Signs of subarachnoid bleeding in several sulci in parietal areas on the right, adjacent to the falx   2
- The hematoma has penetrated into the right lateral ventricle, which is practically obliterated   4
- Choroid plexus in the left lateral ventricle appears normal   1
- There is a midline shift toward the left, and edema surrounds the periventricular white matter on the right   2
- Raised intracranial pressure (obstructed ventricle) and herniation of the brain (edema) can be expected   4

Solution to exercise 9 (p. 70): — 9 Points

Gray and white matter appear well defined on narrow brain windows.

	Level	Width	Gray scale	
	+ 35 HU	80 HU	- 5 HU to + 75 HU	3

CCT sections are normally oriented parallel to the orbitomeatal line, 2

so that initial and follow-up studies can be precisely compared.

2-mm sections at 4-mm increments are acquired through the petrosal bone, 2

then thickness and table movement are set at 8 mm. 2

Solution to exercise 10 (p. 70): — 16 Points

Intracerebral hemorrhage	in early phases hyperdense, often with hypodense peripheral edema	2
Subarachnoid hemorrhage	hyperdense blood instead of hypodense CSF in the sulci and cisterns	2
Subdural hemorrhage	hyperdense crescentic area close to the calvaria, concave toward the cortex, not limited by cranial sutures	4
Epidural hemorrhage	hyperdense, biconvex area close to the calvaria, smooth toward the cortex, always limited by cranial sutures	4
Complications	hemorrhage into a ventricle, CSF flow is obstructed, edema, danger of herniation	4

Solution to exercise 11 (p. 70): — 2 Points

Subarachnoid hemorrhage in children may be visible only next to the falx or in the lateral (Sylvian) fissure.

Solution to exercise 12 (p. 70): — 10 Points

Practice makes perfect!

Solution to exercise 13 (p. 70): — 4 Points

Fracture of the right frontal bone and absent right frontal sinus (the latter is a congenital variation, not a hemorrhage, as indicated by the osseous trabeculae)

Solution to exercise 14 (p. 70): — 8 Points

This was a difficult question. In the left internal jugular vein there is unusual sedimentation of the CM due to slow blood flow. The asymmetry of the jugular veins is not a sign of thrombosis. A left cervical abscess makes the neck muscles appear poorly defined.

Solution to exercise 15 (p. 71): — 4 Points

In this patient the surface subarachnoid spaces are clearly too narrow and the ventricles distended. These signs indicate that CSF drainage is reduced or blocked and there is imminent danger of brain herniation. There is generalized brain edema. A neurosurgeon should be consulted about inserting an intraventricular shunt.

Solution to exercise 16 (p. 71): — 3 Points

It is possible to mistake the subarachnoid hemorrhage around the left frontal lobe as an artifact. The left frontal cortex is outlined by blood. If you did not see any abnormality, return to the chapter about the head.

Solution to exercise 17 (p. 71): — 6 Points

You have of course taken the hint about not giving up too soon; the right medial rectus muscle (47c) is thickened. It is the second muscle to become involved in endocrine ophthalmopathy. If you cannot remember which muscle is affected first, return to page 59.

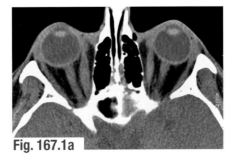
Fig. 167.1a

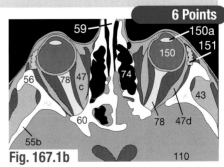
Fig. 167.1b

Solution to exercise 18 (p. 71):

Part of the question was misleading, but this was intentional, and I hope you take it in the right spirit. No fresh intracranial bleeding can be seen in this image **(Fig. 71.4** is the same as **Fig. 168.1).** The abnormality in the left frontal lobe is an area of reduced attenuation representing an earlier hemorrhage **(180)** which has now reached the resorption phase (4 points). The extracranial swelling and bruising in the left frontoparietal area (1 point) is also 2 weeks old. In order to determine the nature of the hyperdense foci, particularly on the right side, you should of course ask to see adjacent images (4 points). The next caudal section **(Fig. 168.2)** shows that these foci are formed by the orbital roofs **(✳)**, the sphenoid bone **(60)**, and the petrosal bone **(✳✳)** (1 point for each). These partial volume effects were discussed on page 51. If you misinterpreted them in the question, take it as a warning and you will be less likely to make this mistake again.

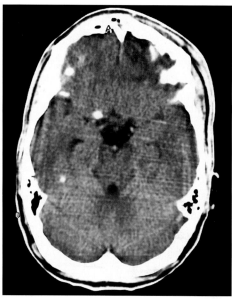

Fig. 168.1a

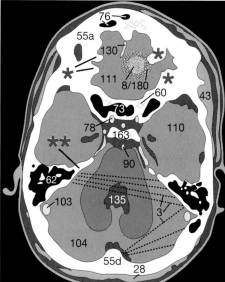

Fig. 168.1b

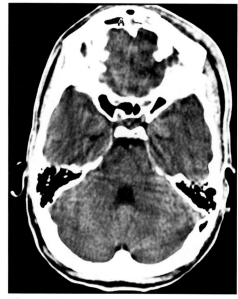

Fig. 168.2a

Fig. 168.2b

Solution to exercise 19 (p. 80):

Compare your checklist for CCT with the one on page 72. As in exercise 1, each item is worth ½ point and the correct sequence is worth 3 points.

Solution to exercise 20 (p. 110):

There is an area of low attenuation due to incomplete CM filling in the azygos vein, most likely because of a thrombosis (2 points). The esophagus is not well defined. There are hypodense lines crossing the pulmonary trunk and right pulmonary artery which are artifacts because they extend beyond the lumen of the vessels (2 points).

Solution to exercise 21 (p. 110):

Did you suggest doing bronchioscopy or biopsy in order to know more about the "lesion"? Then you must revisit the basic rules of CT interpretation. But if you remembered to look first of all at the other images in the series, as for example the one on the right, you will have seen that the "lesion" belongs to the sternoclavicular joint (↖). This is another example of a partial volume effect. There is degenerative change in this joint, but no pulmonary lesion or inflammation.

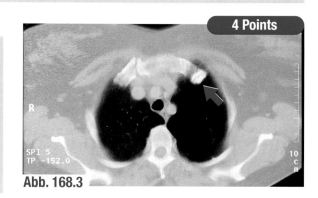

Abb. 168.3

Solution to exercise 22 (p. 110):
The cause of sudden back pain in this patient was the dissection **(172)** of the aortic aneurysm (1 point). At this level, both the ascending **(89a)** and the descending **(89c)** aorta (1 point each) show a dissection flap. It is a de Bakey type I dissection (1 point).

4 Points

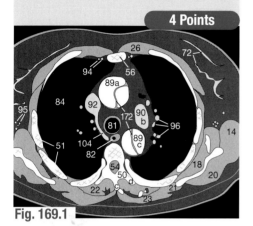

Fig. 169.1

Solution to exercise 23 (p. 110):
This is a case of bronchial carcinoma (the bronchial obstruction is not seen at this level). There is atelectasis of the entire left lung **(84)** (2 points) and an effusion **(8)** fills the pleural spaces (2 points). Did you detect the metastatic mediastinal LN **(6)**? (2 points)

6 Points

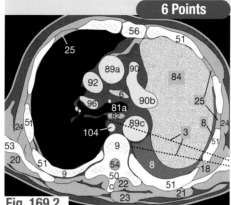

Fig. 169.2

Solution to exercise 24 (p. 111):
The most obvious abnormality is the bronchial carcinoma **(7)** in the left lung. The right lung shows emphysematous bullae **(176)**. CT-guided biopsy of the tumor should be possible without causing a pneumothorax because it has a broad pleural base (2 points).

6 Points

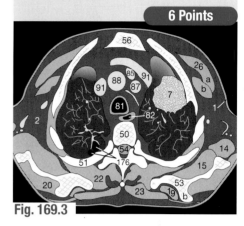

Fig. 169.3

Solution to exercise 25 (p. 111):
The small metal clip **(183)** is a hint that the stomach has been surgically transposed into the mediastinum. The thick-walled structure with the irregular lumen is a part of the stomach **(129)**, not an esophageal tumor. At the moment of data acquisition the stomach was contracting and is therefore not as easily identified as in **Figure 101.2**.

4 Points

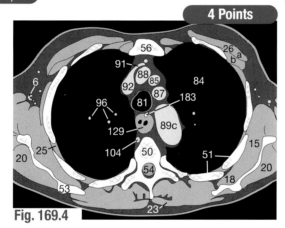

Fig. 169.4

Solution to exercise 26 (p. 111):
You are already familiar with this tragic case of bronchial carcinoma in a young pregnant woman (thus no CM enhancement, see **Fig. 108.2**). The anterior locule of the malignant effusion (3 points) had caused the right lung to collapse (2 points) and was therefore drained. After the fibrin clot had been removed from the catheter the lung was reinflated and the mother's life was prolonged until the birth of her healthy child. Did you notice the metastatic LN in the right axilla? (1 point)

6 Points

Solution to exercise 27 (p. 111):
Perhaps the first thing you noticed was the irregular contour of the diaphragm **(30)** (1 point), but this is a normal finding. The patient was a smoker and had complained of weight loss. You should first ask for lung windows in order to check for metastases **(7)** or primary bronchial carcinoma (5 points).
When a chest is examined, it should become your standard procedure to use both soft-tissue and lung windows **(Fig. 169.5a)**

6 Points

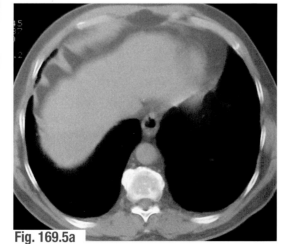

Fig. 169.5a

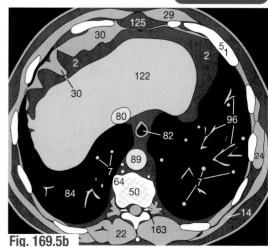

Fig. 169.5b

Solution to exercise (p. 111):

4 Points

These two images show an aberrant branch of the aortic arch: The subclavian artery passes posterior to the trachea and the esophagus toward the right side of the body. You may remember that this anatomic variation was mentioned, but not shown, on page 98.

Solution to exercise 29 (p. 135):   **4 Points**

In addition to the air–fluid levels in the dilated bowel (2 points) associated with an ileus, you should have seen the dilated right ureter anterior to the psoas muscle (2 points). The correct diagnosis is therefore ileus and hydronephrosis. You may recognize this particular case as the same one shown in **Figure 128.2a**, at a slightly more cranial level.

Solution to exercise 30 (p. 143):   **7 Points**

This is a case of left inguinal hernia **(177)** (1 point). There are normal LN bilaterally **(6)** (1 point). Did you identify the femoral artery **(119)**, the profunda femoris artery **(199a)**, the femoral vein **(120)**, the deep femoral vein, and the gluteal vessels **(162)** (1 point each)?

Solution to exercise 31 (p. 143):   **7 Points**

You should have seen the adenoma **(134)** in the right adrenal gland (2 points). For ¹/₂ point each you should be able to name ten other organs. Consult the number legends if you are uncertain.

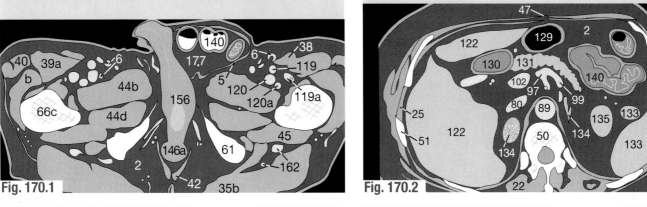

Fig. 170.1

Fig. 170.2

Solution to exercise 32 (p. 143):   **4 Points**

This is indeed a case of situs inversus (2 points). You will also have noticed that the attenuation of the liver **(122)** is abnormally low: fatty liver (2 points).

Solution to exercise 33 (p. 143):   **3 Points**

The question itself will have drawn your attention to the atherosclerotic plaques **(174)** in the common iliac arteries **(113)** (1 point). The left one is part of an aortic aneurysm (2 points).

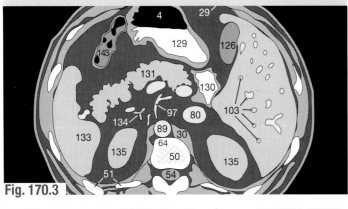

Fig. 170.3

Fig. 170.4

Solution to exercise 34 (p. 143):   **6 Points**

Hopefully you saw the fairly large, irregular metastasis **(7)** in the posterior segment of the liver **(122)** (1 point). Did you also see the smaller, more anterior metastasis? (3 points). The DD may have included an atypical hepatic cyst (1 point) or, for the anterior lesion, partial volume averaging of the falciform ligament (1 point).

Solution to exercise 35 (p. 143):   **5 Points**

The two cysts **(169)** in the right kidney **(135)** are impossible to miss (1 point). But there are also multiple, hypodense lesions in the spleen **(133)**, due to splenic candidiasis (3 points). You may also have considered a rare case of nodular lymphoma or melanoma metastases in the spleen (¹/₂ point each).

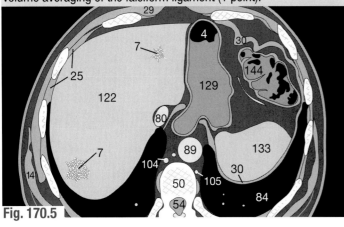

Fig. 170.5

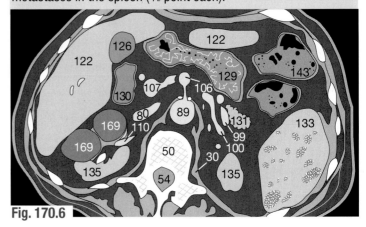

Fig. 170.6

Solution to exercise 36 (p. 144): **6 Points**

Figure 171.1 is the section next to the one in **Figure 144.1** and shows that the hypodense area in the liver is the gallbladder. If you suggested doing anything else, for example aspiration or biopsy, before seeing adjacent sections, take 3 points away.

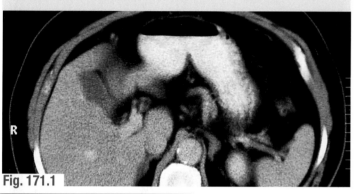

Fig. 171.1

Solution to exercise 37 (p. 144): **5 Points**

You may have thought that the hyperdense foci next to the rectum **(146)** represent calcified LN **(6)** (1 point). However, the lymphatics are so well demarcated because they are still opacified after lymphography (3 points). Did you also notice the atherosclerotic plaques **(174)** in the femoral arteries **(119)** (1 point)?

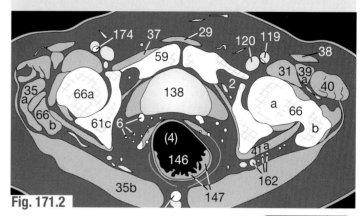

Fig. 171.2

Solution to exercise 38 (p. 144): **3 Points**

You will achieve the most accurate densitometry of a cyst if you select a section without any partial volume effects from renal parenchyma as in **Figure 144.3b** (1 point). Results of measurements in **Figure 144.3a** would be too high (2 points). Since this very case was discussed on page 127, take away 2 points for the incorrect answer.

Solution to exercise 39 (p. 144): **7 Points**

The illustration showed only one metastasis in the right lobe of the liver (1 point) in a case of hepatomegaly (1 point). By using triphasic SCT, additional metastases become visible (2 points). CT arterial portography (3 points) is more invasive than SCT alone, but it demonstrated that the spleen also has metastases.

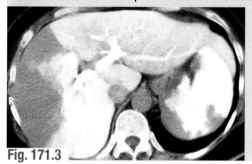

Fig. 171.3

Solution to exercise 40 (p. 144): **6 Points**

For further documentation you should ask to see bone windows (2 points) and of course the adjacent sections (2 points) in order to assess the pelvic fracture. It is also important to determine whether the acetabular fossa was involved (2 points). The fractures of the pubic bones were already visible on soft-tissue windows **(Fig. 144.5)** because the fragments were slightly displaced.

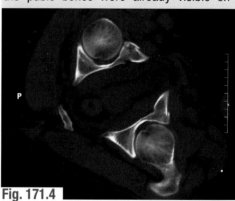

Fig. 171.4

Solution to exercise 41 (p. 145): **10 Points**

If you detected the fresh thrombosis **(173)** in the right femoral vein **(118)**, you get 3 points. Did you also see the synovial cyst **(175)** on the left (3 points)? Your DD may have included a lymphoma, a femoral or inguinal hernia, or a metastasis (1 point each). If you mistook the cyst for thrombosis of the left femoral vein as well, take away 3 points! The vein **(118)** lies next to the cyst.

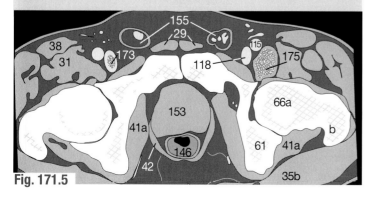

Fig. 171.5

Solution to exercise 42 (p. 145): **7 Points**

Another example of a partial volume effect: the sigmoid colon was only apparently "within" the urinary bladder (4 points). The first thing you should have asked to see was adjacent sections (2 points). You may remember that this case was discussed on page 112 (see **Fig. 112.5a**).

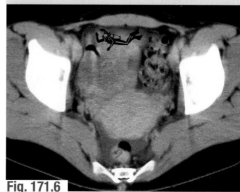

Fig. 171.6

Solution to exercise 43 (p. 145): **11 Points**

The beam-hardening artifacts **(3)** due to drainage tubes **(182)** were a hint that this image was taken shortly after surgery (2 points). The abnormal structures containing gases **(4)** are surgical packs (5 points) placed to control bleeding after multiple trauma. When the patient's condition had stabilized they would be removed in a second operation. Your DD may have included fecal impaction in Chilaiditi's syndrome (2 points) or an abscess with gas-forming bacteria (2 points).

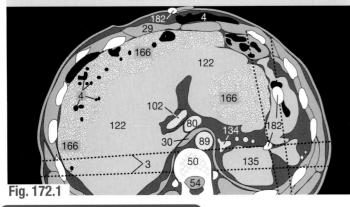
Fig. 172.1

Solution to exercise 44 (p. 145): **8 Points**

You may have thought that **Figure 145.4** shows a gastric pull-through for esophageal carcinoma (1 point) or that the esophageal walls are thickened due to metastases (2 points). However, this was a case of a paraesophageal sliding hiatus hernia (3 points). If you forgot to ask for lung windows, you will not have seen the large right paramediastinal emphysematous bulla (➡) (2 points).

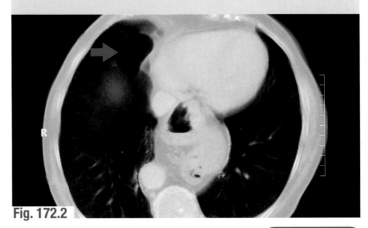
Fig. 172.2

Solution to exercise 45 (p. 145): **11 Points**

In **Figure 145.5** a poorly defined tangential section of a diverticulum of the urinary bladder can be seen next to the rectum on the right side (✶) (5 points). Your DD may have included a pararectal LN (2 points). The irregularities in the attenuation values of the urine are due to CM and the 'jet phenomenon' (2 points each). **Figures 172.3** and **173.4** are adjacent to **Figure 145.5**.

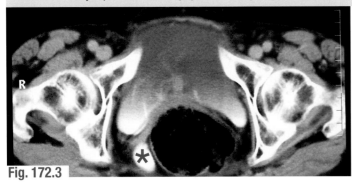
Fig. 172.3

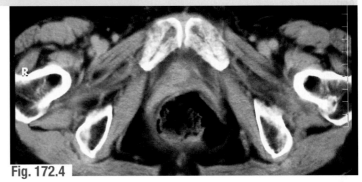
Fig. 172.4

Solution to exercise 46 (p. 145): **4 Points**

The same old problem! The hyperdense (enhanced) C-shaped structure in the pancreas **(131)** in **Figures 145.6** or **172.5** is a loop of the splenic artery **(99)** (4 points). The adjacent sections (c, d, and e) show that the splenic artery can be very tortuous.

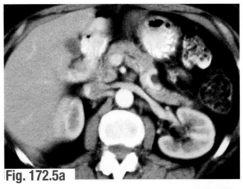
Fig. 172.5a

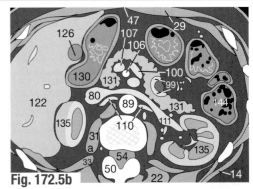
Fig. 172.5b

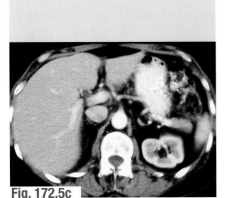
Fig. 172.5c

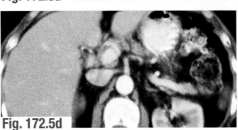
Fig. 172.5d

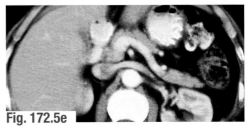
Fig. 172.5e